Put Down the Knife

Michael H. Brisman

Put Down the Knife

A Fresh Look at Adult Brain Surgery

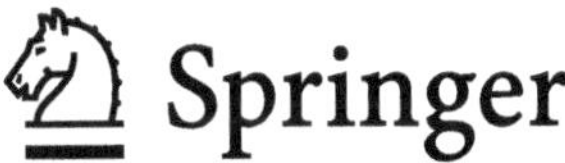

Michael H. Brisman
NSPC Brain and Spine Surgery
Rockville Centre, NY, USA

ISBN 978-3-031-48501-5 ISBN 978-3-031-48499-5 (eBook)
https://doi.org/10.1007/978-3-031-48499-5

This Springer imprint is published by the registered company Springer Nature Switzerland AG
The registered company address is: Gewerbestrasse 11, 6330 Cham, Switzerland

Printed on acid-free paper

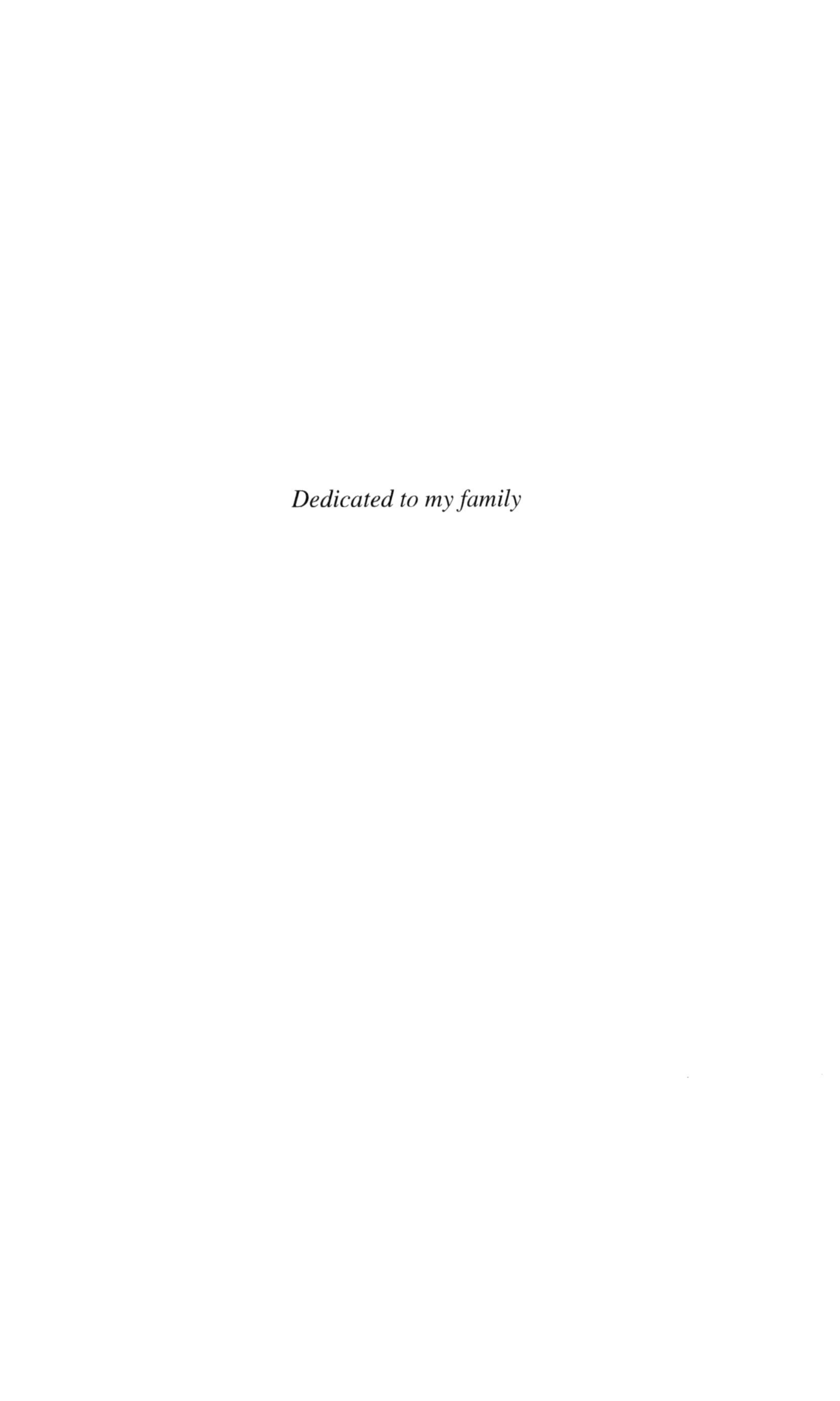

Dedicated to my family

Introduction

Modern adult brain surgery is a very new discipline. While many would consider the fathers of modern neurosurgery to be people like Victor Horsley, Harvey Cushing, and Walter Dandy, they all worked in the early twentieth century, in an era before the creation of equipment that we now consider to be "game changers" in the field of neurosurgery. Only toward the end of the twentieth century did we see such critical advances as the operating microscope, the wide availability of CT and MRI imaging, neuro-endoscopy, stereotactic neuronavigation, stereotactic radiosurgery, interventional neuro-endovascular techniques, and intra-operative neuromonitoring. It is not just that these advances occurred only recently, but it is even more recently that they have become accessible to many neurosurgeons. Furthermore, the scientific evidence for adult brain surgery in this new era is itself extremely new and a work in progress.

I was born into neurosurgery. My father was a neurosurgeon, and I was born in Baltimore while he was doing a general surgery internship at Johns Hopkins, just before he went to do his neurosurgical training at the Neurological Institute in New York. After my full neurosurgical training (pre-medical undergraduate studies, medical school, general surgery internship, and neurosurgical residency), I joined a private practice on Long Island, New York. When I joined the practice, there were only two senior neurosurgeons; at the time I write this book, we have 20 neurosurgeons in our practice. For the past 20 years, I have focused almost entirely on adult brain surgery, with a strong emphasis on trigeminal neuralgia, brain tumors, and stereotactic radiosurgery. I have overseen my group and various regional hospital programs. I have also made a deliberate effort to read the major medical and neurosurgery journals since I started my residency. I believe, like my father, that learning is a lifelong process, and that the purpose of a formal education is to teach a person how to teach themselves.

There is certainly both an "art" and a "science" to the practice of medicine and to the practice of adult brain surgery. Furthermore, there is also a wide range of acceptable practices in regard to adult brain surgery, ranging from the most conservative/minimally invasive options to the most aggressive approaches. I am of the belief that the pendulum in medicine has swung way too far to the "art" side and away from the "science." Furthermore, I believe that given the very high risks associated with adult brain surgery, that the default choice of treatment should be the more conservative/minimally invasive options when possible. This book explores adult brain surgery from a more conservative vantage point.

Acknowledgments

One of my father's favorite stories was when he was first beginning his studies at Harvard Medical School in 1961. His instructor told the class that half of the things they would be taught in medical school would ultimately turn out to be untrue, and unfortunately, they did not know which half.

If I wrote anything in this book that is useful or helpful to people, my accomplishment is because I stood on the shoulders of giants.

If I wrote anything in this book that is objectionable or unhelpful to people, the fault is all mine.

Sometimes you must go public with an idea to push a reluctant organization in the direction you want it to go.

—Nelson Mandela

Contents

About the Author

Michael H. Brisman grew up in Bergen County, New Jersey, and graduated valedictorian from The Frisch High School in Paramus. He received his undergraduate degree with high honors in biology from Harvard University and obtained his medical degree from the Columbia College of Physicians and Surgeons. He then completed a General Surgery Internship and Neurological Surgery Residency at The Mount Sinai Medical Center in New York City, where he was appointed Chief Resident in his final year of Residency. He subsequently joined a private practice neurosurgery group on Long Island, New York, where he has worked for the past 25 years. In addition to maintaining a busy clinical practice, he serves as CEO of his medical practice, NSPC Brain and Spine Surgery.

He is board certified by the American Board of Neurological Surgeons and is a Fellow of the American College of Surgeons. He served as the Chief of Neurosurgery at Winthrop University Hospital (now NYU Long Island Hospital) and serves as the Co-Medical Director of the Gamma Knife program at Mount Sinai South Nassau Hospital. He has served as the President of the Nassau County Medical Society and President of the New York State Neurosurgical Society. He currently serves as a delegate for the Medical Society of the State of New York and the American Medical Association. He specializes in the treatment of trigeminal neuralgia and brain tumors and has treated thousands of patients with these conditions.

About the Author

Part I
General Concepts and Errors in Thought About Adult Brain Surgery

Chapter 1
General Concepts About Adult Brain Surgery

Are there too many surgical operations being performed?

There is reason to believe that the answer is "yes," not just for adult brain surgery, but across the board. For example, there is evidence that some 30% of Medicare patients (American patients mostly over age 65) have at least one surgery in their last year of life [1], and studies have also shown that surgery on frail, elderly patients rarely helps them live better or longer lives [2]. Now one could argue that it would be fairly difficult to test this general premise on the population as a whole. One way would be to stop most, if not all surgery that was being done, and see if it made a difference, but no one would ever agree to such an experiment. But is not that exactly what happened during the 2020 COVID-19 pandemic? Numerous areas throughout America and the world shut down their hospitals for most surgical procedures (and for most standard hospitalizations) for several months straight. The results? The harm? The devastation from people missing their critically needed surgery? The truth is that we did not really see that much harm at all. Of course, there were individual cases presented of the consequences of the missed surgery. But, as a whole, the public outcry for their surgery was really pretty muted. That is not to say that some surgery is not beneficial, but it certainly strongly suggests that a lot of the surgery performed is not really as critical and beneficial (or as urgent) as many people think it is.

As surgeons, we need to start asking with each operation: "Was that operation really absolutely necessary and unavoidable?" and "Was an alternative, less invasive, or nonoperative treatment a reasonable option?"

Why Adult Brain Surgery Is Different

One could argue that the study of adult brain surgery is, in fact, no different than the study of anything else. I would disagree for a few reasons. First, adult brain surgery is arguably one of the highest risk things a person can have done to themselves.

M. H. Brisman, *Put Down the Knife*,
https://doi.org/10.1007/978-3-031-48499-5_1

Second, the risks undertaken in adult brain surgery are undertaken for purely therapeutic purposes. That is, there may be many "risky" things people do, but they are doing them for the enjoyment, or adrenaline rush, or lack of awareness, or some other reason. People accept the risks of adult brain surgery, knowing that there are serious risks, for the sole purpose of achieving some significant improvement in the quality of their lives, or the length of their lives, or both. Third, adult brain surgery, due to transformative advances in just the past 20 years, can be performed with a degree of safety that has not been present before, especially if one considers minimally invasive adult brain surgery alternatives. Fourth, medical advances have also progressed dramatically, such that non-surgical alternatives are often at least as good as surgery.

Major Minimally Invasive Brain Surgery Interventions

The two major categories of minimally invasive brain surgery that have fundamentally changed the way brain surgery is practiced are (1) stereotactic radiosurgery and (2) endovascular neurosurgery. The ramifications of these two techniques on modern adult brain surgery cannot be overstated.

Stereotactic radiosurgery is a super-focused radiation technique that usually involves gamma rays (such as with a Gamma Knife machine) or x-rays (such as with specially modified Linear Accelerators or "LINACs"). This technique can be used for treating brain tumors (both malignant and benign), brain vascular malformations (including arteriovenous malformations, arteriovenous fistulae, and cavernous malformations), and various functional disorders (such as trigeminal neuralgia, glossopharyngeal neuralgia, and refractory tremor).

Endovascular brain surgery is a catheter based technique that can be used for diagnostic cerebral angiography, brain aneurysm coiling and stenting, brain arteriovenous malformation and arteriovenous fistulae embolization, mechanical thrombectomy for stroke, embolization for epidural hematoma and chronic subdural hematoma, pre-resection tumor embolization, carotid stenting, intra-arterial medicine applications for cerebral artery vasospasm, and carotid or vertebral artery sacrifice (for some rare giant aneurysms).

While there are other specialists besides neurosurgeons who will perform these techniques, such as radiation oncologists for stereotactic radiosurgery and radiologists and neurologists for endovascular brain procedures, it is critical for neurosurgeons to remain fully active participants in these two fields. For example, the neurosurgeon who performs radiosurgery should be deciding independently which patients to treat with this technique and exactly how to treat them (obviously with confirmation/concurrence from the radiation oncologist). Furthermore, it is best for the neurosurgeon who specializes in these fields to be fully adept at the "open" brain surgery procedures for the diseases treated by these "minimally invasive" techniques. By fully understanding both the less invasive and more invasive brain surgery techniques, the neurosurgeon can help guide the patient to the optimal choice of treatment.

What Is the Purpose of Adult Brain Surgery?

While the answer may seem obvious, it is surprisingly not obvious to many. The purpose of adult brain surgery should be (1) to "significantly" increase the length of a person's life that is enjoyed at a certain high quality that cannot be achieved by "non-surgical" measures; (2) to "significantly" increase the quality of life that a person enjoys for the same length of time, which cannot be achieved by non-surgical measures; or (3) to "significantly" increase both the length of a person's good quality life and the degree of quality of a person's life, which cannot be achieved by non-surgical measures. As such, these are the only relevant "primary endpoints" for a study that purports to justify any brain operation.

Now one could argue about what constitutes a "significant" increase in life or a "significant" improvement in life, but we should generally agree that this is the purpose of adult brain surgery. Lengthening a life by a few weeks would hardly seem to justify brain surgery; extending by 5 years the life of someone who has a poor and miserable quality of life would also seem to be of dubious value. Furthermore, the burden of proof should be on the brain surgeon to establish that the proposed procedure is likely to dramatically improve length of life, quality of life, or both, and in a manner that could not otherwise be achieved.

General Neurosurgical Insights

While there are obviously many general points to be made on surgery and neurosurgery, I will mention only a few.

- *Primum non nocere*—first do no harm (an ancient concept in medicine).
- Good surgeons know how to operate, better ones when to operate, and the best when not to operate [3].
- If there is a question about seeing the patient, see the patient. If there is a question about getting a CT scan, get the CT scan. If there is a question about putting in a ventriculostomy, put in the ventriculostomy. And always be nice to the nurses (Dr. Ronald Brisman).
- Incidental findings ("incidentalomas") are usually benign and usually best left alone or observed.
- Often the only surgery that was really necessary was the surgery to fix a complication from the first operation.
- The best way to minimize the length of a patient's hospital stay (other than selecting the least invasive treatment option) is to tell the patient when they are expected to be discharged. For example, I will tell my microvascular decompression and transsphenoidal patients that they will need to stay overnight in the hospital. This has helped tremendously in having these patients agreeable to being discharged the day after surgery.

- Very few people really need brain surgery, and those who do will usually be best served with a minimally invasive procedure. Said another way, "the best operation is usually no operation," and "less is usually much more" when it comes to adult brain surgery.
- If a medical intervention or operation is considered to be "controversial," there is a good chance that the medical intervention or operation is not going to be helpful.
- The best way to avoid a serious complication is to limit surgery, particularly in eloquent or high-risk areas, unless absolutely necessary.
- The more complicated and riskier an operation is, the less likely it is to be helpful.
- Surgeons often completely underestimate the importance of the appropriate "timing" of surgery. Many operations that are helpful will only be so if performed in a very specific time frame. For example, sometimes a brain operation must be performed fairly quickly, and often the more significant the symptoms and the more rapidly the symptoms have developed, the more quickly surgery will need to be performed to be beneficial. Conversely, sometimes the surgeon must wait before performing an operation, either because time is needed for proper medical clearance and optimization, because a further work-up is needed, or because one must allow anticoagulants to be fully eliminated from a patient's system.
- A surgeon should not aggressively dissect tumors, or other things, that are stuck to cranial nerves or critical blood vessels. If the abnormality is benign, it does not matter, and if the abnormality is malignant, it also does not matter. Residual abnormalities can usually be treated in other ways, such as with stereotactic radiosurgery or standard radiation therapy.
- If an inexperienced person has a complication, the most likely cause of the complication is the person's inexperience.
- The longer the list of patient complaints, the less likely the problems can be fixed with surgery.
- Having a surgical trainee (resident or fellow) perform part of an operation necessarily increases the risk of that operation, particularly if the trainee is not being directly supervised by an attending surgeon.
- A surgeon should never be the only one to know bad news. If there is a serious medical issue, or serious diagnosis, or any other serious problem, it is critical that it be communicated promptly to the appropriate people, whether that is the patient, family member, chief resident, attending physician, chief of service, nursing supervisor, hospital administrator etc. This is a particularly critical concept for physicians in training, like residents and fellows. Prompt communication of serious matters that arise in complex systems (like hospitals) is critical for trust and safety.
- The best surgical outcomes occur when the surgery is performed by an experienced attending surgeon, with an experienced operating room team, during regular weekday hours.
- After a neurosurgical residency or fellowship, neurosurgeons still require a significant amount of proctoring and oversight from more experienced neurosur-

geons. Many more errors are made by neurosurgeons in the first few years out of training than subsequently.

- Surgeons cannot optimize their performance if they do not actively engage in the non-surgical management of potential surgical patients and the non-surgical management of patients after surgery. Furthermore, lengthy follow-up is often needed for the surgeon to fully appreciate their own successes and failures. The full extent of surgical benefits and complications is often not appreciated for a long time.
- The base of a scalp flap should be at least 1.5× as long as the depth. This is important to maintain proper vascularization to the flap and to avoid the risk of ischemia to the deepest portion of the flap.
- Fibrin sealants are associated with an increased risk of complications [4], so they should only be used if absolutely necessary.
- SURGIFLO should not be used near the ventricles as intraventricular application can cause hydrocephalus.
- Great caution should be used in manipulating a patient's neck once they are under anesthesia. Many people, particularly older patients, have underlying cervical spine disease, and aggressive manipulation can cause a spinal cord injury.
- Hyponatremia in patients with acute brain disease is usually caused by cerebral salt wasting syndrome (and is associated with euvolemia or hypovolemia). Sodium replacement (oral or intravenous) along with gentle hydration should be used for gradual correction. Blood sodium level correction must be gradual to avoid causing central pontine myelinolysis.
- A good surgeon is a humanitarian who cares not only about what happens to their own patients, but to other people as well. They have great compassion, and they have a great fund of knowledge. They keep up to date on advances in their field, and they have good judgment.
- A good surgeon never forgets their worst complications.

Who Should Be the "Captain of the Ship"?

The phrase "captain of the ship" is often invoked in the medical setting, with the question being, who should be the ultimate decision maker for a given medical decision.

The most appropriate person to make decisions about adult brain surgery is the brain surgeon. Obviously, one cannot proceed with any decision to operate or not operate without support of the patient and others, but ultimately, the person who should have the most insight into the issue is the surgeon.

It is not reasonable to suggest that some other physician should be making this decision. It is even less reasonable to suggest that medical extenders, like nurse practitioners or physician assistants, should independently be making any such decisions (for these or any other major medical issue).

A real threat to such proper decision-making is the decreasing ability of the neurosurgeon to function as part of an independent private practice. While it is not critical that all neurosurgeons work in a private practice for them to be able to make the best decisions for their patients, it is necessary that such practice be a viable option. Absent this, brain surgeons, like other physicians, will just feel compelled to make decisions that please their employers.

Four General Classifications of Brain Surgery

One might consider breaking down brain surgery procedures into four types of categories as listed below:

1. Clearly indicated, performed with few complications;
2. Clearly indicated, performed with high complications;
3. Not so clearly indicated, performed with few complications;
4. Not so clearly indicated, performed with high complications.

Category 1 procedures, ideally, would make up most of the adult brain surgery procedures that are performed. These are clearly indicated procedures that are performed well with few complications. Unfortunately, I would contend that there are many procedures performed that would fit into categories 2, 3, and 4.

Category 2 procedures will often be justified with the argument that the case was clearly indicated, and complications necessarily happen at a certain rate, without really questioning whether the surgeon or circumstances of the surgery might have contributed in some way to the complications that occurred and suboptimal outcome.

Category 3 cases are often deemed acceptable because doctors and hospitals are under pressure to produce a certain surgical case volume, so, even if the surgical indications were somewhat questionable, the case will be tolerated due to the low rate of complications and side effects.

Category 4 cases will also often be overlooked if the patient was likely to do poorly anyway. Category 4 cases performed in otherwise young and healthy people are least likely to be tolerated but may still get a pass from other doctors and administrators if the frequency of these events is not too high for that particular surgeon or that particular hospital.

The Major Flaw in How Most Neurosurgeons View Adult Brain Surgery

There are many misconceptions that neurosurgeons and others currently have in regard to adult brain surgery, but they all come down to the following main error: There is a consistent gross underestimation of the risks of adult brain surgery, and there is a consistent gross overestimation of the benefits of adult brain surgery. This single error leads to many "open" procedures, generally craniotomies, being performed, when a less invasive alternative or no procedure at all would have been preferable and yielded better results.

A recent study [5] gives some sense that this conclusion is correct. Their prospective study of neurosurgery patients included 2258 patients undergoing brain surgery. Of these, some 24% had complications, of which 57% were graded as "severe." And even this number of complications is likely dramatically understated as various major categories of complication were not even considered, like pain, anxiety, depression, subtle permanent deficits, and inability to return to work. Furthermore, there is real evidence that hospital stays are much riskier than most people realize. For example, a recent large study of 2809 consecutive hospital admissions found at least one adverse event in 23.6% of admissions, with about a third of the adverse events being "serious" [6].

I will deal separately with many different standard adult brain surgery topics, but it is important to first understand what might be the sources of confusion in general, before I discuss each topic in particular. These sources of error are numerous.

Chapter 2
Errors in Thought About Adult Brain Surgery

Here, I will explore specific errors in regard to adult brain surgery decision-making and the pertinent review of published scientific studies.

"This Is How I Was Trained"

This is one of the most common arguments that a neurosurgeon will use to justify the decision to perform adult brain surgery and the specifics of the operation they have chosen to perform. But the flaw in this argument is clear. Just because someone else was doing something a certain way does not prove or establish anything. It may be that the teacher or professor was doing something that was the second-best possible way of treating a certain problem, for whatever reason. It may be that the instructor was doing something the best possible way, at that time, but a few years later, a better treatment became available or became more apparent. Oddly enough, people will make this argument 10, 20, or even 30 years after they were trained, even though the discipline has rapidly changed since then.

"I Have Seen Patients Do Well After This Surgery"

This argument again is not definitive evidence. The patient may have done well without the surgery. The patient may have done well because of something else besides the surgery. The patient may have done well with a much more limited operation. The patient may have done well with some less invasive treatment that did not involve surgery. The patient may have done well because of a placebo effect. The patient may have done well immediately after surgery, but 3 months later may have had serious problems. Observing that one or more patients do well after an

M. H. Brisman, *Put Down the Knife*,
https://doi.org/10.1007/978-3-031-48499-5_2

operation in no way establishes that that operation or any operation was clearly necessary.

"The Patient Wanted the Surgery"

In this scenario, the proposed justification for a particular brain operation is that the patient themselves "wanted" the brain operation. First, people only really want a brain operation that is likely to help them. Second, people will usually only agree to an invasive brain procedure if they are presented with no reasonable alternative. Third, the patient is no expert on brain surgery. As such, a surgeon should not justify an operation with the argument that "the patient wanted the surgery."

A variant on this concept, for patients who cannot make their own decisions, like debilitated patients or minors, is "the family wanted the surgery." Obviously, this is just the same argument and not in itself a valid reason to proceed with surgery.

"The Family Wanted Everything Done"

This incorrect argument arises, usually in an emergency situation in which the extremely unfortunate patient is unable to make their own decisions, and brain surgery is performed with the justification that "the family wanted everything done." It could also be that the family wants "everything done" because they believe this is what the patient would have wanted. But this is just a variation on the theme of "the patient wanted the surgery." Clearly, the family would want brain surgery for their loved one "if there was evidence that it would help." But the family is in no position to know that answer, even with a thorough internet search. It is the brain surgeon's job to inform the family about whether surgery is or is not indicated.

This is not to say that different patients may indeed have different preferences, and some may be more willing to live with significant disabilities than others. Nonetheless, it should be the brain surgeon who is guiding most of the decision-making and informing the family of what surgery would or would not generally be helpful for their unfortunate family member. A surgeon should not justify an otherwise pointless operation with the argument that "the family wanted everything done."

"We Have Nothing to Lose by Operating"

This argument is usually made in some desperate situation in which surgery would not normally be advisable, and the surgeon reasons that "we have nothing to lose by operating." These scenarios include both the suddenly devastated but hopeless patient, as well as the patient with chronic severe disability with a very poor quality of life. But this same argument could be used to justify any operation in any hopeless situation. The issue should be "is there evidence that there is clearly something to be gained from the operation," not simply that the situation is so dismal that an operation will not make matters any worse. It is also very common in these hopeless situations that a few days after the brain surgery, a "serious" discussion takes place with the family and palliative care is instituted. Clearly, this discussion could have just as easily taken place before the surgery and avoided a pointless operation.

"Surgery Is Not Clearly Worse Than the Alternatives"

There are circumstances in which this may well be the case. There may well be no study or definitive evidence that surgery is worse than other known alternatives. But is that really an adequate justification to operate on the brain? Given the obvious risks involved, the real standard for performing adult brain surgery should be strong evidence that the procedure is clearly better than other alternatives, not just that it is not clearly worse.

"We Were There Anyway"

This argument involves an operation that may well have had legitimate indications, which then becomes coupled with other procedure(s) for different purposes or of a more prophylactic nature performed in the same general vicinity with the justification that "we were there anyway." These "secondary" procedures would not have been justified on their own and only add risk to the primary operation. Yet many surgeons will often justify such procedures with the argument that since we were already working in that area, adding some other procedure was theoretically acceptable. This is usually not the case, and such additional work just adds risk to the primary surgery.

"The Brain Issue Was the Presenting Problem, Therefore We Should First Perform Surgery on the Brain"

This argument is just not correct. For example, a neurosurgeon is consulted to evaluate a patient who had a seizure, and a CAT scan demonstrates what looks like brain metastases. An MRI confirms this suspicion, and the neurosurgeon operates on one of the tumors to make the diagnosis. Again, the fact that the brain problem was the presenting problem in no way argues that it should be surgically addressed first or at all. The more reasonable course would have been to start the patient on a seizure medicine (like Keppra), and some steroids if there were edema (like dexamethasone), and to perform a CAT scan of the chest, abdomen, and pelvis. If a large lung mass was found, a bronchoscopy might well yield a diagnosis without any brain surgery, and the brain metastasis or metastases could be treated with radiosurgery or standard radiation.

"Brain Surgery Should Be Performed Because There Is Brain Edema or Mass Effect"

This argument usually reasons that there is brain edema or mass effect, and that if this is not promptly addressed with surgery, these features will progress and lead to serious neurological symptoms or brain herniation and death. This argument is also frequently not correct. For example, brain metastases will often have edema yet rarely will benefit from open surgery. Steroids and radiation/radiosurgery are the mainstay of management for brain metastases. The steroids can often be quickly tapered after radiation treatment.

"We Need an Invasive Diagnostic Procedure"

This is generally a call for a cerebral angiogram or other procedure that carries small but real risks. Again, while such procedures may well have been "standard" years ago, now, in the age of CT, MRI, CTA, CTV, MRA, and MRV imaging, these invasive diagnostic procedures are often not necessary. And the risk of angiography is real, potentially very serious, and not zero.

"We Need Tissue"

This assertion is made very frequently as a justification for brain surgery, when, in fact, there is rarely a need for "tissue" in order to care for the patient. Most of the time, the diagnosis is clear from the imaging or history (such as a known history of active systemic malignancy). In some select cases (e.g., some gliomas), it may be appropriate to obtain diagnostic tissue if that can safely be done. But that is the exception. The request for "tissue" is often made by non-surgeons, and the brain surgeon will claim justification for operating because these other specialists wanted the surgery performed.

"The Tumor Board/Trauma Board/Stroke Board Recommended Surgery"

This may involve the request for an unnecessary diagnostic procedure or the unnecessary obtaining of lesional "tissue," but it can also involve more extensive procedures such as brain tumor removals, brain hematoma evacuation, decompressive craniectomy, and so on. The obvious problem here is that these boards are filled up mostly with people who do not specialize in neurosurgery and are just not in the best position to make recommendations about brain surgery. Usually, most members of these boards have never met the patient and have no neurosurgical training. Operating merely to satisfy such committees will not improve outcomes.

"We Need To Do This Procedure to Satisfy Certain Volume Requirements"

This is one of the most cynical arguments. For example, an argument is made that the hospital needs a certain number of annual mechanical endovascular thrombectomies for stroke to maintain its stroke center designation, so, even though a particular patient is probably not a good candidate, the surgeon or interventional neuroradiologist should perform the procedure anyway, for the good of the hospital. Or the hospital needs to put in a certain number of intracranial pressure monitors (or "bolts") to maintain its trauma center designation, so the surgeon should put such a brain monitor in a patient, even though it is unlikely to be helpful, for the good of the hospital and the overall program. It is obvious why brain surgery to satisfy this and only this criterion is not likely to be helpful.

"This Is What Was Said at a National Conference"

National conferences are held periodically, and certain neurosurgeons will present on a brain surgery topic they are experienced with. But any such presented recommendations cannot be determined to be "the best possible recommendations" simply because they were given such a forum for presentation.

Surgeons who are doing things a certain way will be much more likely to invite other surgeons to speak publicly who share their views, and surgeons who do speak publicly will also want to present their work in the best possible light. Suffice it to say, that an attendee at a given conference who subsequently performs a recommended procedure is in no way guaranteed to see comparable results.

"This Patient Is a Very Important Person (VIP)"

In some cases, a surgeon will justify an operation with the argument that this particular patient was an unusually important person, whether because the patient (or the patient's relative) was a doctor or nurse or hospital administrator, or politician or famous person, and so on. The surgeon seems to acknowledge that had the person been a "regular" person, they would not have operated, but given the special status of this individual, they thought that operating was somehow the best thing to do. The suggestion seems to be that a more important person or their family will be more appreciative of what appears to be a more aggressive approach in a circumstance when such surgery would not otherwise be offered. Again, this argument is unsound. Furthermore, a VIP and their family will likely be more appreciative of an honest assessment and treatment based on scientific evidence than a brain operation that is otherwise unnecessary.

"This Is How Everyone Is Doing Things"

This argument proposes to justify a particular indication for brain surgery by suggesting that many or most other people are performing the same operation for similar indications. It may well be that if a lot of people are performing a particular operation for a particular reason, it is a good idea. But it certainly is not definitive evidence, and the reality is that brain surgery indications have been rapidly evolving. As such, one cannot argue that some operations must be appropriate just because lots of other surgeons are performing such an operation.

Now the reality is that every possible aspect of every possible intervention can never be studied, and it is not unreasonable to point to what most reasonable people believe about something. But such "general sentiment" cannot override solid scientific data and is not strong evidence in itself.

Chapter 3
Errors in Thought About Published Studies on Adult Brain Surgery

The argument that "published studies support this operation" is often not valid. This is the most commonly used argument to justify adult brain surgery and is usually the biggest problem. As such, the numerous errors in thought that occur in relation to published studies need to be addressed in detail.

The Biases of the Authors

The authors are often motivated to publish and particularly to publish "positive" studies (studies that show that surgery was helpful). If they publish good results, it will improve their reputation, referrals, and their careers. If they publish poor results, it may harm their reputations. Doctors with poor results are much less likely to publish their outcomes than doctors who can portray good results.

The net result is not surprising. Major neurosurgery journals are filled with positive results, positive studies, and positive outcomes. Most studies suggest that surgery is highly effective and that risks are minimal. There are few studies that put a negative spin on any type of brain surgery. The real risks and downsides to brain surgery are easily lost in reading the published literature.

The Biases of the Editors and Reviewers

The editors are also often biased toward positive results and more aggressive interventions. This is not completely surprising. The neurosurgeon editors, like the neurosurgeon authors, love their profession and want to believe that there are more and more helpful things that neurosurgeons can accomplish in the operating room. As

M. H. Brisman, *Put Down the Knife*,
https://doi.org/10.1007/978-3-031-48499-5_3

such, editors are much too willing to allow the author to draw an overly optimistic conclusion about surgery that is not clearly substantiated by the data.

Mistaking "Statistical Significance" with "Clinical Significance"

Often, a study will proclaim that a certain brain surgery procedure should be done because their study showed that something was "statistically significant." This can be very deceptive. Certainly, we want our studies to show statistical significance, that is, a demonstration that the data is sufficient to show that the results are unlikely to have occurred by chance. But it depends on what is being measured.

For example, a certain brain operation is found to extend life, and this is found to be statistically significant. But we really need to know a lot more. Was the extension of life of a "clinically significant" amount? Was life extended by only a few weeks or 10 years? Was the extension of life a good quality of life or life in a very incapacitated state? Unless the statistically significant finding related to a major extension of a good quality life, or a major improvement in the level of quality of life, or both, it does not really matter at all, and the conclusion would be not to do that operation.

In summary, of course statistics matter, but only insofar as they tell us that patients are really better off.

Looking at the Wrong Endpoints

Often, a study will suggest a procedure should be done based on a statistically significant improvement in a less critical or "secondary endpoint." For example, a study will show that patients who receive a certain brain operation are 25% less likely to die of stroke, and therefore, the procedure should be offered. But this endpoint is not what patients really care about. Now it certainly makes sense, if one is doing a procedure that we believe would help people by reducing stroke risk, to look at the subsequent rate of stroke. But that alone is not enough to recommend the procedure. One needs to demonstrate, again, that there is significant improvement in length or quality of life. If, for example, the patients had a 25% decrease in the likelihood of stroke but had no improvement in quality or length of life for whatever reason, the surgery would be pointless. What if these patients ended up with an otherwise unappreciated 40% increase in the rate of fatal heart attack within the first year of the surgery? The point is that it is just not enough to say that the rate of stroke was decreased to recommend the surgery. We need to know that the patients were really better off overall. Another common example is looking at endpoints such as "progression free survival" and "length of survival" and "30-day mortality" (which are all fine to look at), but without looking at what really matters most, which is to what extent was a good quality of life extended by the treatment.

Drawing Conclusions That Do Not Follow from the Study's Results

In these cases, the study's conclusion simply does not follow from the reported results of the study. For example, the study will show something, statistically significant or not, and then draw the common conclusion that such brain surgery "may have a role" or such brain surgery "should be studied further." In fact, these are frequent conclusions of clinical brain surgery studies no matter what they show. There is never a recommendation to just stop doing such and such brain operation. The careful reader must always assess if the conclusion really follows from the data presented.

Incorrect Assumptions About Lack of Proper Follow-Up Data

Frequently, a study will appropriately want to look at what happened to people over time after surgery. It is appropriately recognized that the benefits or lack thereof cannot always be appreciated immediately after a brain operation. The problem is that usually it is difficult to get appropriate follow-up for all the patients. Some patients move away, some patients are unhappy and stop following up with that doctor, and that is all fine. It would not be fine, however, to assume that these patients had results similar to those of the remaining patients. Such an error is also known as "attrition bias" and is a form of "selection bias." A patient who is "lost to follow-up" may well be lost to follow-up because they died, or became incapacitated, or were unhappy with their surgery with that doctor. One needs to assume that patients who do not respond to follow-up questions may well have done much worse than those patients who were willing to complete follow-up visits and surveys. As a result of assuming that non-responders are similar to the entire cohort for which data exists, the results tend to skew toward a much better result than what likely exists.

Assuming That Published Data Is Representative of Typical Results/Not Recognizing the Selection Bias of Published Reports

This error assumes that published results are representative of the results that other surgeons can expect. This is not the case for several reasons. First, the person who publishes their results is likely more experienced at that operation than the average surgeon. Second, the author often wants his or her results to look as good as possible, so likely frames them in as positive a light as possible. Third, the published samples are not representative. For every surgeon who publishes results with a certain very high success rate and a certain very low complication rate, there are likely many more surgeons who have much lower success rates and much higher complication rates who would just not publish that particular data. As such, a surgeon cannot assume that their results will match results described in published articles.

Minimizing or Ignoring Significant Complications

The studies that are published will often entirely dismiss serious complications and problems that patients have after brain surgery. Patients will sometimes have long-term pain in the incision area. They may have long-term headaches. They may just feel weaker than they used to be. They may have some bothersome numbness, or dysesthesias, or other neurological deficit that just never completely goes away. They may not ever be able to return to work. Their vision or hearing or sense of smell may never return to the state it was before. They may forever feel somewhat off balance. They may have ongoing tinnitus or dizziness. They may suffer from new depression or anxiety. They may require new medicines that cause serious side effects.

All these problems are usually left out of surgeon follow-up visit notes and just considered "an expected result of such surgery," but anyone who is in practice and performs brain surgery knows that many people have real and significant long-term negative consequences to brain surgery that are often just brushed off. A published study may show a post-op MRI that looks very good, but all sorts of real problems for that patient never get mentioned. For many patients, there is some real truth to the saying that "when the air hits your brain, you're never quite the same."

Overstating the Benefits of Surgery

This again happens very frequently, for various reasons, and is related to many of the errors mentioned already. The benefit may be something that is offset by other problems that develop. The benefit does not translate into real increase in quality of life or high-quality survival. The authors do not adequately consider the other less invasive alternatives that might have provided an equally satisfactory outcome. This problem happens all the time.

Not Properly Factoring in Placebo Effects

Most people do not realize how strong a placebo effect can be. In fact, if people are told a certain medical intervention will help them, surprisingly, some 20–30% of patients or family members may say that they think the procedure was helpful. As such, even when many patients or patient families report postoperative improvement, there may be no objective improvement at all. This just reflects the fact that patients may feel improvement from even a totally non-effective treatment, and family members often will believe there is an improvement, or want to report that there is an improvement, even when there really is none. The reality is that many people will feel very happy and lucky if they have the good fortune to have brain surgery and not end up dramatically worse.

Resorting to Meta-analyses

These really have little role in the justification of adult brain surgery. The concept here is that while numerous studies may have, in themselves, shown no real benefit to a certain brain operation, maybe if many such studies were looked at in aggregate (whether with a "meta-analysis" or a "pooled analysis"), it might be possible to demonstrate some minor statistically significant result. But this is not appropriate in this context. If one is looking to identify if the tiniest of changes is occurring as a result of a certain action, then a meta-analysis may make sense. But when it comes to adult brain surgery, given the magnitude of the risks and downsides, there is really no justification to perform a given operation if the benefit is so subtle that it can only be detected in a meta-analysis.

There is also a real problem if the studies selected for inclusion in the meta-analysis were not chosen in a completely random manner—obviously if a person gets to select which studies to "pool together," data can be swayed in any direction one pleases.

This all is not to say that a meta-analysis might not provide some other insights, like the full range of all the complications that might occur from such a procedure. But such assessments really have little role in establishing the usefulness of a brain operation.

The Call for Endless Studies

This error occurs when, despite numerous similar studies showing that a given procedure is not helpful, there is insistence that there is more information needed and that the procedure should still be done and investigated ad infinitum. Common examples of these are the nearly endless studies that have been done trying to demonstrate that it is generally beneficial to remove intracerebral hemorrhages or to perform craniectomies for trauma patients. Though study after study has shown that these practices are not generally beneficial (though of course there may always be rare exceptions), each study seems to call for yet more studies and suggest the matter can never be resolved conclusively.

Not Recognizing That the Operation(s) Was No Better Than Less Risky Alternatives

This is also surprisingly common. An author will present the most high-risk, novel, unique surgical approach to a problem without considering that not doing that operation may have yielded just as good a result. This is the same problem really as just lacking a proper control group for the study.

Not Recognizing That a Component of a Necessary Operation May Be Unnecessary

While it may be the case that a particular brain operation may in fact be necessary and helpful, there may still be parts of that procedure that were not necessary or helpful (and just added unnecessary risk to the procedure). For example, a study that looked at young patients who underwent emergent evacuation of large subdural hematomas and concurrent placement of an intracranial pressure (ICP) monitor might show good results compared to a control group that received no intervention at all. But it may be that the ICP monitor did not add anything to the results, and there would have been the same number of patients with good outcomes, or even more with good outcomes, had the surgeon just removed the subdural hematoma and not placed the ICP monitor. The fact that brain surgery is helpful does not mean that every component of the procedure was helpful.

Incorrectly Relying on Other People to Determine If Surgery Was Necessary

Often the entire basis for the surgery is "failure of non-surgical treatment." Unfortunately, this determination is usually left to people who are not experts in the area of interest and not in a position to adequately make this determination. For example, a study may say that surgery was performed in patients who had failed medical management. The question becomes: "Failed medical management according to whom?" Ultimately, the conditions for which a brain surgeon would consider operating are specialized enough that the brain surgeon must be able to confirm that the patient has truly failed other options.

Reliance on Post-Hoc Analyses

This maneuver occurs after a study is completed, usually unsuccessfully, and the authors attempt to salvage the study with some subsequent retrospective analysis of a small subgroup of the treated patients that perhaps did show some benefit from the surgery or intervention. The problem here is that this subgroup often cannot be identified in advance, and therefore, while the analysis serves to justify yet additional studies, these are also likely to be futile. For example, the MISTIE III trial [7], a study of 506 patients with moderate to large intracerebral hemorrhages treated with or without placement of a surgically placed catheter with subsequent placement of a clot dissolving agent (alteplase) until there was less than 15 cc of clot left (if possible), showed no difference in the two groups. This was yet another study on evacuation of intracerebral hemorrhage that showed no benefit to surgical intervention. After the study, a subgroup was identified that had less than 15 cc of blood left (58% of the total), and in those cases there was a very modest (10%) improvement in the rate of good functional outcome. But there would be no way, in advance, to know which were the patients for whom that volume would have been achievable in, and regardless, the benefit even in those cases was a very slim one. Nonetheless, surgeons who operate on intracerebral hemorrhages took this study, which again concluded that such patients should not be operated on, to do just the opposite and continue to operate on such patients, in the hope of providing some ever so slight benefit. And as we have already explained, adult brain surgery should really only be performed in cases in which the benefit is significant and clear.

Biases Due to Outside Funding

Nothing ruins the reliability of a study more than outside funding. This so taints the study that this alone puts any positive results into question. When a company is paying for the study of brain surgery using a tool they produce, or using a drug they produce, or using an implant they produce, the pressures on the authors to demonstrate a beneficial result increase dramatically. The authors will do anything to spin the results in some positive way. As such, until the results are reproduced by someone who is not being funded by that company, they should be considered very uncertain.

Studies That Are Ended Early

Suspicion should be raised when a study is artificially ended early. Such an event should be rare, and only in the case that the evidence was so overwhelming that it would be unethical not to immediately stop the study and offer or stop offering one of the treatment options. But, again, this should rarely be the case. Presumably, if the study was being conducted at all, there was real doubt regarding how obvious something was. It is far more likely that the person or persons controlling the study wanted to quickly declare victory when there was none and prevent a full and complete evaluation that might not have shown the benefit they wanted to show. This is just another form of "selection bias," in this case, preferentially using data that was collected earlier in the study. A study that ended early but is still used to justify a treatment, particularly an invasive one, is a red flag.

Studies Created to Justify a Preferred Conclusion: "Self-Serving Studies"

In the age of the scientific method, for anything to be considered valid, it must have some "scientific" study that confirms its accuracy. That has not changed the natural human goal of self-interest and of advocating for matters that would be advantageous to that individual but not necessarily to others. So regardless of whether something is correct or not, it is highly likely that someone will generate a study to show that it is correct if that serves someone's interests. This practice is so common that before even reading a study, the careful reader will ask themselves: "Why did the author(s) publish this?" Since so many publications have become in some way "self-serving," it follows that many studies are also not completely reliable.

Post-Hoc Ergo Propter Hoc Errors

This is the classic error of concluding that because event Z happened after event W, that event Z was caused by event W. One must consider numerous other possibilities. W and Z may be completely unrelated, and the two events could just be a coincidence. W could be causing event Y, and Z may just happen to be associated with Y. W could just happen to be associated with event X, and X is what is actually causing Z. Event V might be causing both W and Z, so it might just appear that W and Z were related. And so on. It is critical to consider all the possible reasons why one event might follow after another.

Studies with Impossible Results

In these studies, the outcomes are just too good to be true, or the complication rate is just too good to be true. Someone who reads the scientific literature should not have to check their common sense at the door. Skepticism is appropriate for all studies that seem to show results that seem too incredible to believe, with benefits that seem unbelievably spectacular, and complications that seem to be nearly nonexistent. The real issue is, can real-life people, using the same techniques, match these incredible results?

Now we have to acknowledge the existence of incredibly talented surgeons. These are people who genuinely perform at levels that far exceed those of most people. Nonetheless, when presented with seemingly spectacular results, we should have some skepticism until the results are duplicated in other clinical studies.

The Dismissal of a Large Good Study That Rejects Numerous Weak Studies

One strong study is worth 100 weak ones. Periodically, a large, well-done study will be published that clearly rejects the findings of numerous prior weaker studies or some commonly held belief. Often, this superior study will be politically inconvenient and will demonstrate that a long-held belief about the benefits of a particular surgery is actually incorrect.

A good example of this issue was when the ARUBA study was carried out [8]. Neurosurgeons had been reporting for years their excellent results for excising unruptured brain AVMs. However, they had inadequate controls and likely poor patient follow-up. In the ARUBA study, patients with unruptured brain AVMs, in which neurosurgeons felt surgical intervention was an option, were randomized to intervention versus nothing. Expert neurosurgeons treated unruptured AVMs with various surgical interventions, and some AVMs were left untreated. Within a relatively short time, due to the high rate of complications in the treatment arm, it became obvious that the patients who were just left alone did far better, on average, than those who received operations. While some neurosurgeons were quick to dismiss this large, well-done, prospective study as somehow flawed, the point is that what can seem like a well-executed brain operation with an acceptable complication rate can still be worse than other options and thus not worth doing at all.

The Study by an Author Who Is Not Familiar with the Alternative Treatments

This practice is just a subset of author bias. These are studies that purport to assess the difference between two main procedures or treatment options. In these studies, the author tries to demonstrate the superiority of Surgery A (which the author performs regularly) over less invasive Surgery B and non-surgical option C (which the author does not offer and has little familiarity with). Invariably, these studies demonstrate that the procedure that the author regularly performs is somehow a better choice or an excellent choice when compared to the alternative options, even though the author has never offered the other options and has little knowledge about them. The weakness of these studies is obvious.

Studies with Inadequate Sample Size

Studies that have a small number of patients involved must always be viewed with suspicion, just as studies with large numbers of patients are much more convincing. Even when small sample sized studies purportedly show a "statistically significant result," such results could be altered with the erroneous assessment or consideration of even a few cases. Obviously, the extreme example of this is the "case report" in which only one case is assessed. These may still be worthwhile if the outcome is dramatic and the case is rare. Nonetheless, small studies must always be considered with some real healthy skepticism.

Studies with Inadequate Follow-Up

Many good or bad effects of brain surgery, or any medical treatment for that matter, may not be fully appreciated right after surgery or by 30 days. In fact, in the early postoperative periods, patients may focus only on one aspect of their circumstances and are also often on multiple medicines, including steroids and opiates, that may seriously confound the true benefit or lack thereof of the surgery that was performed.

It is also true that it is challenging to collect long-term data on patients. Nonetheless, studies with short follow-ups need to be viewed with skepticism.

Discrediting of Studies by Discrediting the Authors

This is an example of the ad hominem logical fallacy, in which an attempt is made to rebut an argument by discrediting the author of the argument rather than addressing the argument or study or data itself. An excellent study may be performed that seriously challenges long-held beliefs, but people will reject it simply because of who wrote it or where it was performed. For example, people will argue that a study done by doctors from another country is not as reliable as studies done by doctors in our country. Now this may or may not be the case, particularly if the other country was using inferior equipment or technique for some reason. But the routine dismissal of studies simply because of who performed them is not legitimate.

Incorrectly Concluding That Non-inferiority Is Validation

A published study will demonstrate that two treatments have fairly similar outcomes, or at the very least that one more invasive treatment is not definitively inferior to some other less invasive treatment, and then conclude that both options remain equally reasonable to perform. This is not the reasonable conclusion. To justify a more invasive intervention, the standard should be a clear demonstration that the more invasive intervention was clearly the better choice, not just that it was not clearly the worse choice.

For example, consider a study that shows that some brain operation is not clearly inferior to just taking some well-tolerated medicine. This would most certainly not be evidence that both brain surgery or medication were equally reasonable alternatives. To the contrary, this study would strongly suggest that the medication option would be the better choice.

Part II
Specific Conditions for Which Brain Surgery Is Considered

The focus in this section is on which patients with various conditions are likely to benefit from brain surgery, and which surgery is likely to be most helpful. Of note, while proper surgical technique is certainly necessary for optimal surgical outcomes, even the best technique cannot make up for faulty surgical decision making. Furthermore, while general rules for surgery can be stated, every rule has its exceptions, and a good surgeon will sparingly operate on cases which may be "exceptions" to the usual rule. This is not unreasonable because knowledge on these matters is rapidly evolving. I have also inserted some of my own cases as illustrations in this section.

Chapter 4
Brain Hematomas

Epidural Hematoma

These are caused by trauma, often with an injury to the middle meningeal artery. Often, these are relatively minor traumas, and the patient may present with a relatively normal exam, even if there was an initial loss of consciousness. There usually are no significant accompanying contusions. These patients can deteriorate very quickly due to the arterial nature of the bleeding.

If these hematomas are small, they can be observed, and this usually includes a repeat head CT within a few hours, with frequent repeat images after that. ICU admission is required. If there is enlargement, but the hematoma is not so large that it must be removed, or if the initial hematoma was intermediate in size, endovascular middle meningeal artery embolization may stop the bleeding and avoid the need for craniotomy [9]. For large epidural hematomas, surgical evacuation with craniotomy should be performed as quickly as possible and can be lifesaving. Craniotomy is necessary to properly evacuate the hematoma and to identify and cauterize the bleeding blood vessel (see Fig. 4.1).

M. H. Brisman, *Put Down the Knife*,
https://doi.org/10.1007/978-3-031-48499-5_4

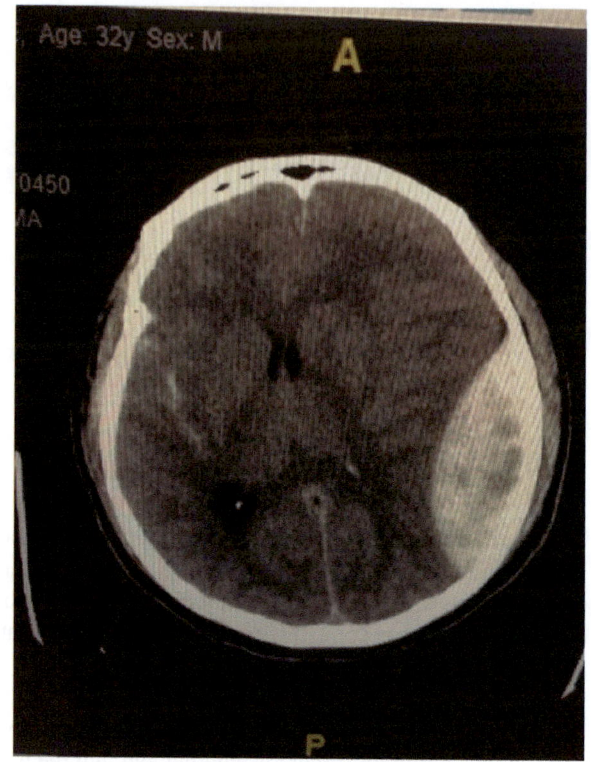

Fig. 4.1 This is a 32-year-old man who was found in the street having been assaulted. There was evidence of head trauma. Upon arrival in the emergency room, the patient was very lethargic and nonverbal. Head CT without contrast showed a large acute left parietal epidural hematoma with significant midline shift. The patient underwent an emergency left parietal craniotomy with evacuation of the hematoma. Over the next few days, the patient made a complete recovery

Subdural Hematoma: Acute

Acute subdural hematomas are usually due to trauma and usually due to venous bleeding. They are more likely to be seen in middle-aged and older patients. In rare cases, these can occur spontaneously, caused, for example, by a ruptured aneurysm or vascular malformation. The traumas that cause acute subdural hematomas are often severe, and associated brain contusions and diffuse axonal injury (DAI) are common. Often, these patients have significant neurological findings on exam from the moment of the injury.

If the subdural hematoma is small and not causing much mass effect, ICU observation with interval CT scans is appropriate. In younger patients, a medium-sized acute subdural may cause shift and mass effect and symptoms and may warrant emergent evacuation. If the subdural is large, immediate evacuation with a craniotomy may be lifesaving. That having been said, evaluation of the overall situation is always necessary. If the subdural is accompanied by numerous other contusions, or the patient is unlikely to make a reasonable recovery for other reasons, no surgery may be best. It is not uncommon for elderly comatose patients to undergo evacuation of their acute subdural hematomas, only for the surgeon to have a "serious" discussion with the family just days later about the hopelessness of the situation. These discussions can just as easily take place before the surgery and avoid a pointless operation.

Sometimes surgeons will also evacuate an acute subdural hematoma and "leave out the bone flap" at the time of surgery. In these cases, the surgeon either discards the bone flap, stores it in the subcutaneous tissues of the abdomen, or stores it in a freezer. This is rarely helpful, and this practice just creates the need for an additional major surgery to repair the skull defect and the numerous added complications of a missing bone flap [10]. Even in cases in which there was some brain swelling due to underlying edema or contusions, it is usually possible to close the skull with a large piece of dural substitute (like Dura-Guard) and a large piece of titanium mesh. The mesh, being much thinner than the bone, already allows for a good amount of brain expansion. Further decompression can sometimes also be achieved with a ventriculostomy, especially if the ventricles are enlarged.

Evacuation of acute subdural hematomas is also sometimes accompanied by placement of an intracranial pressure monitor. This is also not clearly helpful or any more helpful than just getting frequent head CT's to confirm there are no further bleeding sources that require surgical evacuation.

In summary, a moderate to large acute subdural hematoma in an otherwise salvageable patient should be treated with emergent craniotomy, and such surgery may result in a good recovery.

Subdural Hematoma: Chronic

In most cases, these result from minor head trauma, especially, in the elderly. Small subdurals form vascularized membranes, which can then rebleed, and the subdural can thus increase in size, usually over several weeks to months. Chronic subdural hematomas can also result from more serious head trauma, which causes a known acute subdural that then liquefies over weeks. Chronic subdural hematomas must be distinguished from subdural hygromas, collections of cerebrospinal fluid in the subdural spaces, that can sometimes occur after head trauma, and generally require no treatment.

A chronic subdural hematoma that is small can be observed with serial CT scans over several weeks. A medium-sized subdural might also be observed and may regress with time (see Fig. 4.2). Medical management with oral tranexamic acid (TXA) will often eliminate the chronic subdural hematoma [11, 12]. Neuro-endovascular embolization of the middle meningeal artery is also very successful in causing the subdural hematoma to resolve [13, 14]. For larger subdural hematomas, depending on circumstances and symptoms, either medical management with TXA, the middle meningeal artery embolization, or burr hole drainage of the subdural can be considered, though in a stable patient, TXA management and the embolization are less invasive and can also be effective. TXA and embolization can also be successful for patients with chronic subdural hematomas in which there is some mass

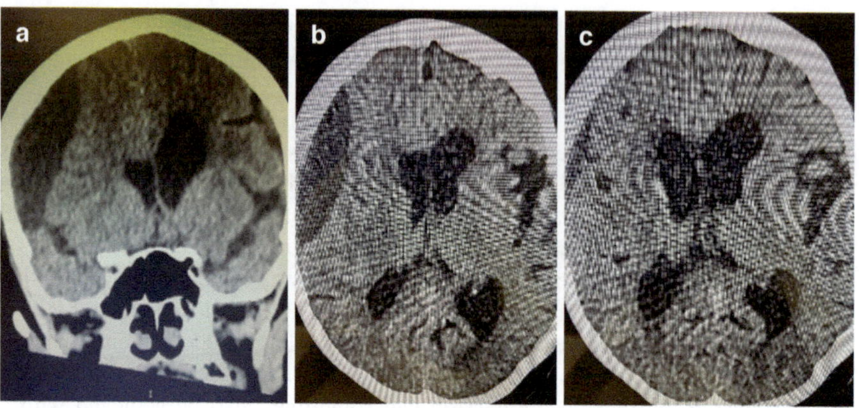

Fig. 4.2 This is a 75-year-old woman who had hit her head several weeks earlier and developed some headaches. Head CT demonstrated a moderate sized right subdural hematoma with some mass effect (**a**: coronal and **b**: axial CT). She was neurologically intact. She wanted to be treated conservatively. She was followed closely with clinical examinations and images. After a few weeks, repeat CT images showed the subdural hematoma had almost completely resolved on its own (**c**: axial CT)

effect or midline shift if there are minimal clinical symptoms (see Fig. 4.3). Because it is less invasive, the medical management or the embolization approach should be preferred when feasible, instead of the open drainage. For patients with significant symptoms and for rapidly deteriorating patients, burr hole drainage should be performed. A bedside twist drill craniostomy drainage under local anesthesia can be performed as well, such as with the subdural evacuating port system (SEPS). Infrequently, craniotomy may be necessary to properly drain a subdural, especially if there are multiple loculated membranes. The inner membrane should not be peeled off the pia of the brain as this may induce seizures and is not necessary for complete resolution of the hematoma. In open surgical cases, a subdural drain for 1–2 days also seems to reduce the risk of re-accumulation of blood. A ventriculostomy drain placed carefully in the subdural space can be used for this purpose. Extra care should be taken to make sure the drain is being placed in the subdural space and not in the brain parenchyma.

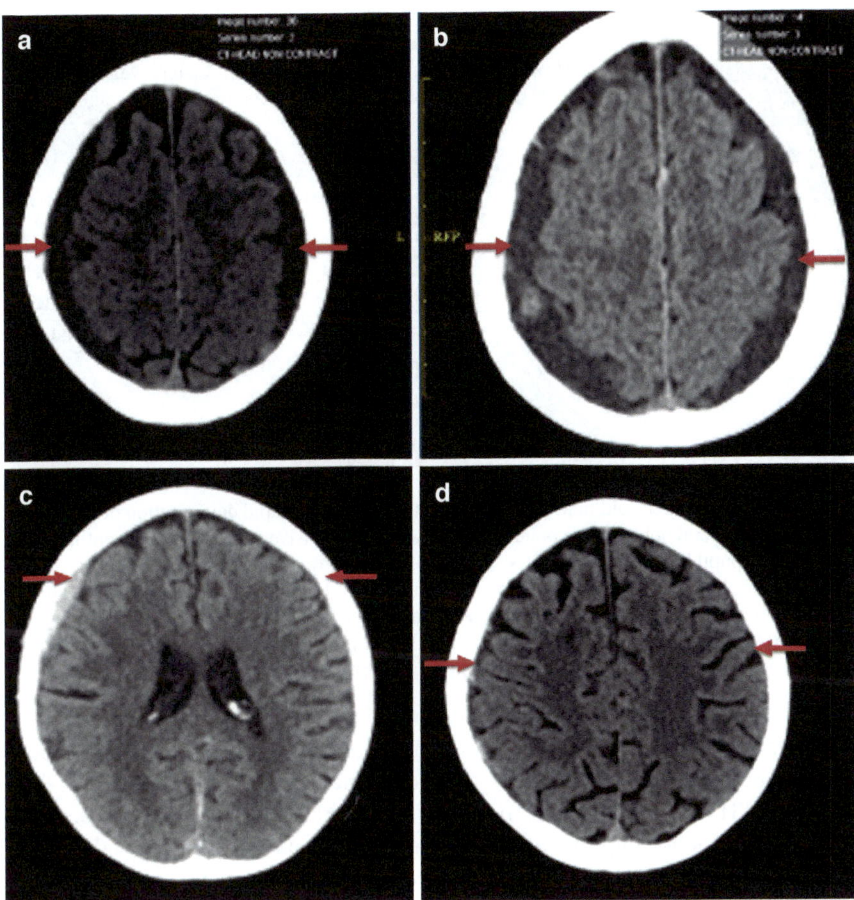

Fig. 4.3 This is an 80-year-old woman who experienced a minor head trauma. She also had CLL and thrombocytopenia. Six weeks later, she had headaches and dizziness and a CT showed bilateral chronic subdural hematomas (**a**). Four weeks later, the hematomas were enlarging with the development of mild sulcal effacement (**b**). Bilateral middle meningeal artery embolizations were performed. One week after embolization, the subdural hematomas were markedly reduced in size (**c**). At 10 weeks post-embolization, the subdurals were nearly gone (**d**)

Intracerebral Hematoma

These can occur for a variety of reasons, including hypertension, amyloid disease, trauma, tumors, and aneurysms. The symptoms will vary depending on the size and location of the bleed.

Numerous studies have been conducted on the possible benefits of surgical evacuation. These studies have considered standard open evacuation, evacuation through smaller cortical incisions, evacuation through small ports, evacuation with stereotactic guidance, evacuation via an endoscope, and evacuation via a stereotactically

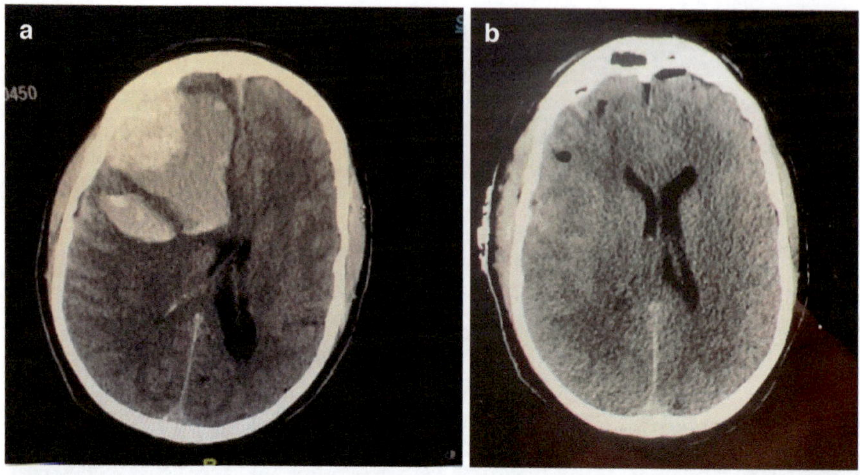

Fig. 4.4 This is a 67-year-old man who presented to the ER with rapid deterioration of neurological exam over several hours, to the point where he was unresponsive and placed on a ventilator. He blew his right pupil in the ER. Head CT showed a large right frontal intracerebral hemorrhage, with perhaps an origin from a superficial region abnormality (**a**). Head CTA was negative. Patient was taken for emergent right frontal craniotomy and evacuation of the bleed. Second CT shows a good postoperative evacuation of the hematoma (**b**). Final pathology showed a brain AVM. Over the next several weeks, the patient made a nearly complete recovery, with only very subtle deficits

placed catheter that would infuse thrombolytics and drain the subsequently liquefied hematoma. What these studies all show—including STICH [15], STICH II [16], STITCH [17], and MISTIE III [7]—is that surgical evacuation of intracerebral hematomas does not improve the percentage of patients who survive with a good quality of life (at least not that could be measured in a statistically significant manner). Nonetheless, this remains one of the more common brain operations performed.

One question is: Are there ever cases in which surgical removal of an intracerebral hematoma would be of value? The answer is "yes," but such cases should be very rare (see Fig. 4.4). One should exclude cases, such as aneurysm ruptures or hemorrhagic tumors, in which open surgery might otherwise be appropriate for other reasons. There is a general thought that such bleeds that might actually benefit from surgery would more likely be in a younger, healthier person, who seemed to still be viable, with a moderate to large bleed, on the non-dominant side, preferably far frontal, and preferably close to the surface. It would be reasonable to conduct a study to specifically investigate the benefits of removal of far-right fontal intracerebral bleeds in otherwise viable patients who are rapidly deteriorating. Regardless, there are a very small subset of such cases in which surgical evacuation is justified, but again, such cases should be very rare.

Intracerebellar Hematoma

These are most commonly caused by hypertension, but less common causes are possible. Current teaching suggests that there are some patients with cerebellar hematomas who will benefit from surgical evacuation. This excludes patients with small hematomas (say under 3 × 3 × 3 cm) who will likely recover on their own. This also excludes patients with very large hematomas (say over 5 × 5 × 5 cm) who will clearly do poorly no matter what. This also excludes intervention in those patients who are viable but develop acute hydrocephalus secondary to their cerebellar hematomas. A ventriculostomy is appropriate here (in an otherwise viable patient) and can enable a good recovery.

So the issue remains as to whether patients with "medium-large" sized cerebellar hematomas benefit from surgical evacuation independent of the need for ventricular drainage. There are some very large recent studies that really call into question this premise, in particular, studies of Kuramatsu et al. [18] that included 6580 patients and Singh et al. [19] that included 2062 patients. Both studies showed no difference in the rate of good outcomes in the patients who underwent surgical evacuation of the cerebellar hematoma versus those who did not.

As such, surgery for intracerebellar hematomas, like surgery for intracerebral hematomas, is likely rarely helpful, though such operations are frequently performed. There are isolated unusual circumstances that might suggest surgery be performed, particularly in a younger patient with a bleed limited to one cerebellar hemisphere, but this should be the exception. The benefits of such surgery for the majority of patients remains very unclear.

Intraventricular Hematoma

These can occur secondary to brain parenchymal bleeds of any kind that rupture into the ventricle secondarily or bleeds that start and remain intraventricular. In viable patients with acute hydrocephalus from an intraventricular bleed, there is certainly a role for emergent placement of a ventriculostomy drain and possibly, subsequently, a permanent shunt, if needed. However, there is no good evidence that surgical evacuation of the hematoma, whether by traditional craniotomy, craniotomy via a port, endoscopic evacuation, or evacuation performed through the ventriculostomy after administration of thrombolytics—such as was studied in the CLEAR III trial [20]—improves the percentage of patients who will have a good functional outcome.

Chapter 5
Brain Vascular Disease

Brain Aneurysm: Ruptured

Brain aneurysms, which may be single or multiple, usually occur as an isolated phenomenon, but rarely can be associated with polycystic kidney disease (a genetic disorder), brain AVMs, or endocarditis.

A brain aneurysm that has ruptured is at high risk for re-rupturing. The re-rupture rate is about 20% in the first 2 weeks and about 50% in the first 6 months. Furthermore, some of the treatments for vasospasm, such as hypertensive therapy and intra-arterial papaverine, are much riskier if the aneurysm is not secured. For these reasons, a ruptured aneurysm in an otherwise viable patient should be treated in a timely fashion, ideally within 24 h of presentation.

Brain aneurysms can be treated by endovascular "coiling" or by craniotomy and "clipping." The coiling procedure is much less invasive and morbid and therefore should be the procedure of choice in almost all cases. The randomized controlled ISAT trial of 2143 patients showed that patients with ruptured aneurysms had significantly better clinical outcomes when they underwent endovascular coiling of aneurysms instead of craniotomy and clipping [21]. In the rare case in which a ruptured aneurysm cannot be coiled, clipping would be appropriate. When an anterior circulation aneurysm must be clipped, the use of neuronavigation can help avoid the frontal sinus, which is well worth avoiding if possible (in this and other frontal craniotomies). Technical keys to these cases, when needed, are early establishment of proximal arterial control and, upon clipping, preservation of parent vessels.

M. H. Brisman, *Put Down the Knife*,
https://doi.org/10.1007/978-3-031-48499-5_5

Brain Aneurysm: Unruptured

The indications for intervention are much less clear here. For most unruptured aneurysms, the annual risk of hemorrhage is likely around 0.05–0.1% per year (ISUIA study, 2621 patients at 53 centers [22]). This is consistent with the known rate of brain aneurysm in the population of about 3–5% and the known annual rate of brain aneurysm rupture. The annual risk tends to be on the higher side, about 0.5–1% per year (1) for aneurysms that are 7–10 mm or larger in size; (2) for posterior circulation aneurysms; and (3) for aneurysms in patients with multiple brain aneurysms who have already ruptured another brain aneurysm [23]. Coiling can be an effective treatment option for unruptured aneurysms [24], and the best case for treatment might be an unruptured aneurysm that meets one of these three criteria and is amenable to coiling. The indications for open surgery for unruptured aneurysms are unclear but, if indicated at all, would likely be for one of the above scenarios in which coiling was not possible. Of note, the risks of serious complications from craniotomy for clipping an unruptured brain aneurysm are not insignificant, and likely in the range of 15–17% [22].

The rare unruptured aneurysm that presents with symptoms needs separate consideration. One special case is that of a posterior communicating artery (PCOM) aneurysm that presents with an acute third nerve palsy. Such an aneurysm should be promptly coiled (or clipped, if coiling is not possible) to avert an impending rupture. Also, giant aneurysms that present with symptoms due to thrombosis might be candidates for endovascular treatments.

The benefits for open surgery for unruptured aneurysms are often greatly overestimated, and the complication rate for such surgery is greatly underestimated.

Brain Arteriovenous Malformations and Arteriovenous Fistulae (AVM/AVF): Ruptured

These vascular anomalies are thought to usually be congenital, with a small percent being acquired lesions. If these present with a hemorrhage in a viable patient, they should be treated if possible. Very small brain AVMs and brain AVFs that can be "embolized for cure"—treated so as to completely eliminate the nidus or fistula—should be embolized. Also, if there is an associated aneurysm that has ruptured, then prompt embolization or coiling of that aneurysm would be appropriate. AVMs that cannot be completely embolized, and that are not extremely large, can be effectively treated with appropriate radiosurgery equipment, such as Gamma Knife [25] (see Figs. 5.1 and 5.2). For Gamma Knife, the preferred dose is 20–24 Gy to the 50% isodose line, depending on the size and location of the AVM/AVF. Certain larger lesions can sometimes be treated with radiosurgery in stages. (Radiosurgery results are better when the lesion is not embolized first.) Also, the AVM nidus is often not as large as people think and may well be amenable to radiosurgery treatment.

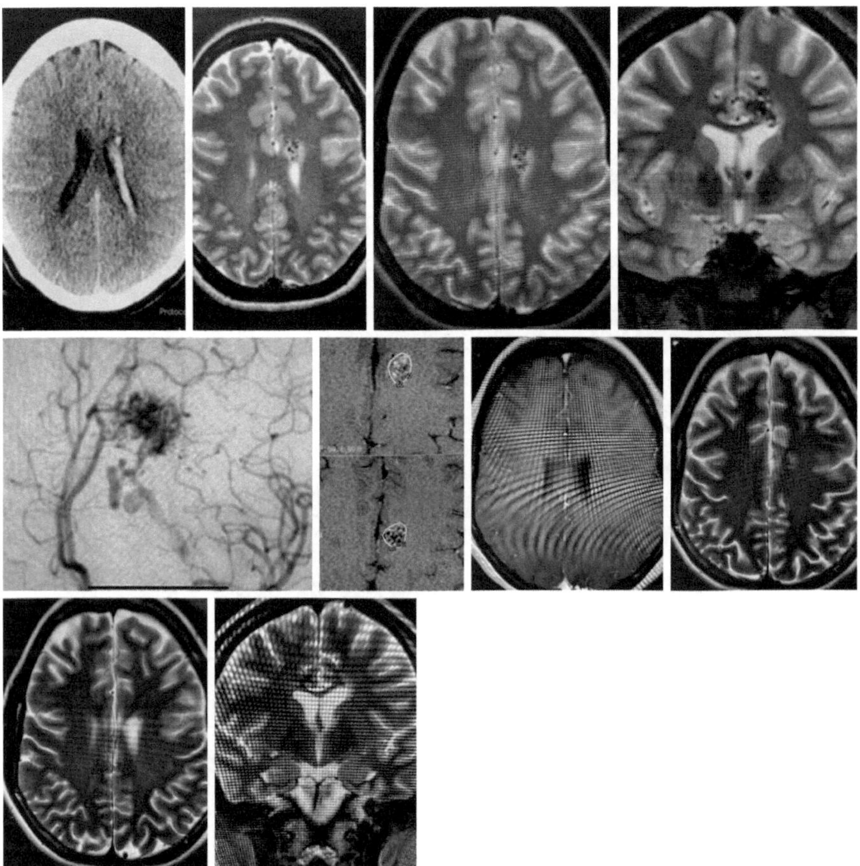

Fig. 5.1 This is a 25-year-old woman who presented with a sudden severe headache found to have an acute left intraventricular hemorrhage (**a**: axial CT image). MRI demonstrated a deep left frontal AVM extending into the left lateral ventricle (**b**, **c**: axial T2 weighted MRI; **d**: coronal T2 weighted MRI; **e**: lateral cerebral left carotid angiogram). The patient fully recovered from the bleed and subsequently underwent Gamma Knife treatment (**f**: axial T1 postcontrast images from the day of Gamma Knife treatment). MRI images 1.5 years after treatment show the AVM is gone (**g**: T1 postcontrast axial MRI; **h**, **i**: T2 weighted axial MRI; **j**: coronal T2 weighted MRI)

Certain lesions, however, are so large that no treatment can reasonably cure the abnormality. If the lesion cannot be completely embolized, and the patient is young and healthy, and the lesion is small and superficial, in non-eloquent cortex, and can be mostly embolized, then open surgery can be considered. It should be rare that a patient with a ruptured AVM or AVF is offered open surgery, over embolization, radiosurgery, or observation only. The complication rates for surgical removal are much higher than are generally appreciated.

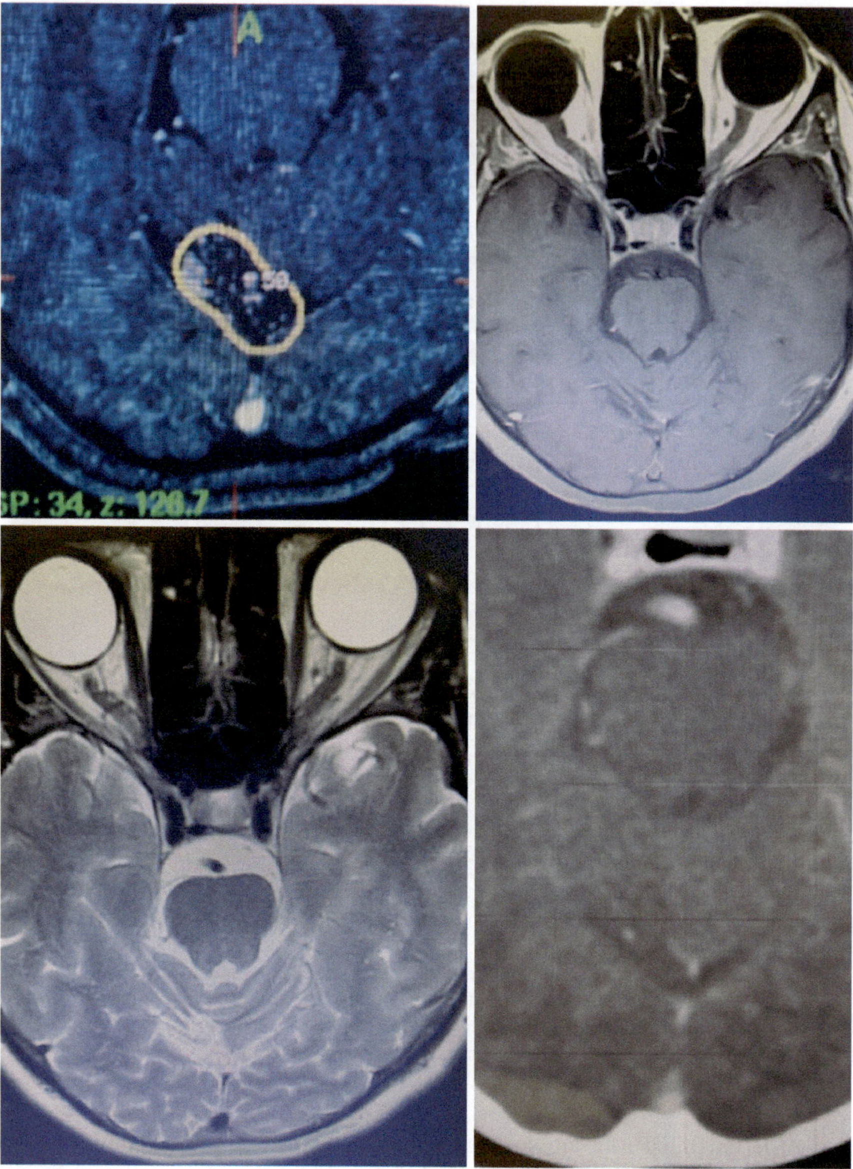

Fig. 5.2 This is a 40-year-old woman who presented with a severe headache and a small bleed from a posterior fossa AVM (upper cerebellar vermis) in her fifth month of pregnancy. She fully recovered and delivered a normal baby. Subsequently, she underwent Gamma Knife treatment (**a**: axial T1 postcontrast images on the day of treatment). She had no subsequent problems, and her follow-up images were showing that the AVM was starting to resolve. She was then lost to follow-up and returned 19 years later to get a check up on things. Follow-up images (**b**: axial T1 postcontrast MRI; **c**: axial T2 weighted MRI; **d**: axial CTA) showed complete resolution of the posterior fossa AVM

Brain AVM/AVF: Unruptured

An unruptured brain AVM/AVF is at lower risk of hemorrhage than a ruptured AVM/AVF. The ARUBA trial [26] looked at patients with unruptured brain AVMs that were thought to be "treatable" and compared those patients who were treated in any manner to those who were not treated. The study showed that the complication rate in the treated group was so high—and so much higher than what surgeons themselves usually reported—that they were expected to never be justified in light of the natural history. Another study showed similar results [27]. However, these studies did not substratify the treatment groups and did not look at, for example, Gamma Knife treatment only versus "no treatment." As such—given the extremely safe profile for Gamma Knife and the real risk of these lesions—treatment with Gamma Knife is likely the best option (see Figs. 5.3 and 5.4). For AVM/AVFs that are tiny that can be cured with embolization alone, this may be performed instead. For AVM/AVFs that are very large, observation only is appropriate. Craniotomy is not clearly helpful. Again, if there were a case in which it might help, it would be for a young, healthy patient, with a very small AVM/AVF, on the surface, in a non-eloquent region, that could be mostly embolized prior to surgery.

Cavernous Malformations: Symptomatic

Most often, when cavernous malformations do cause symptoms, it is because of a small hemorrhage, particularly in a lesion that occurs in an eloquent region. Less commonly, these can present with seizures.

As most symptomatic brain cavernous malformations occur in deep and eloquent locations, an appropriate first line treatment option is usually Gamma Knife [28]. It is rare that patients will require craniotomy. Due to the location of these lesions, surgery is usually high risk and is not clearly better than the alternatives.

Cavernous Malformations: Asymptomatic

These should almost always be left alone. One could, however, argue that for a cavernous malformation in or by an eloquent region, clearly enlarging over time, Gamma Knife would be an appropriate treatment.

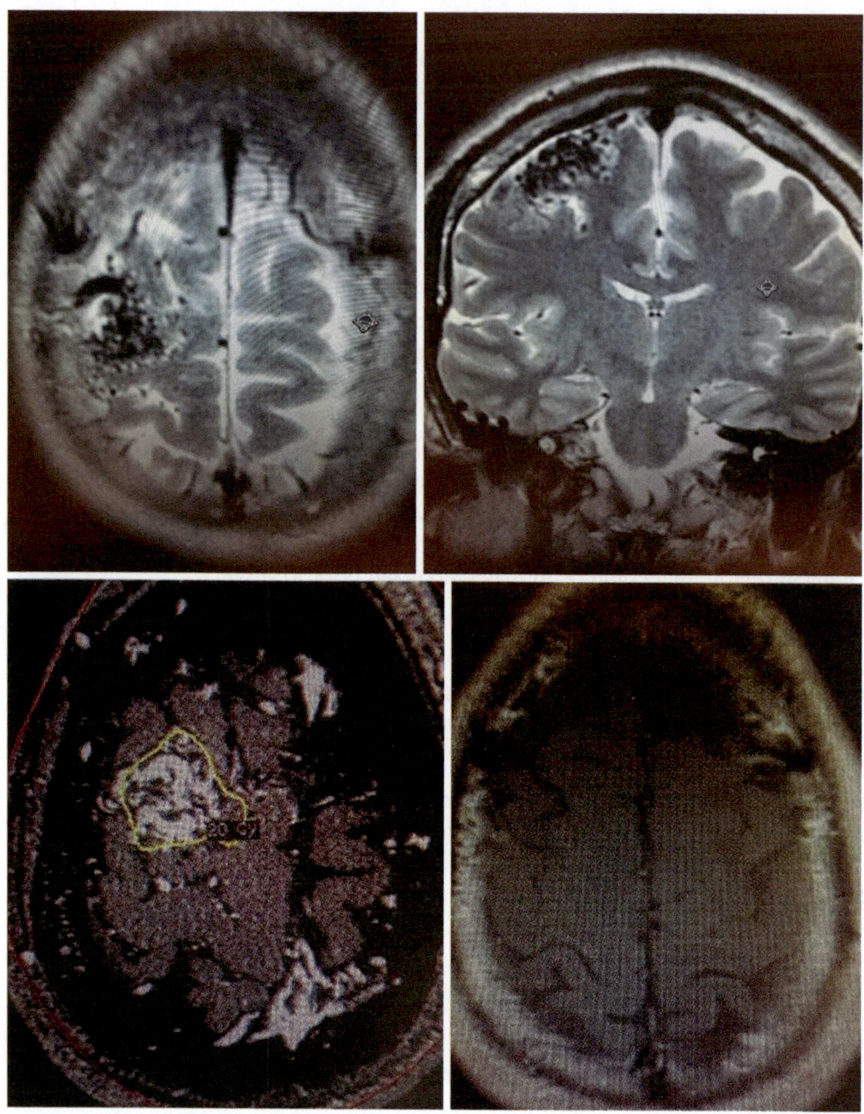

Fig. 5.3 This is a 28-year-old man who presented with headaches and was found to have a 2.5 cm right frontal AVM (**a**: axial T2 weighted MRI; **b**: coronal T2 weighted MRI). Gamma Knife was performed (**c**: day of Gamma Knife treatment, postcontrast T1 axial image). Three years later the AVM is gone (**d**) and he has no symptoms

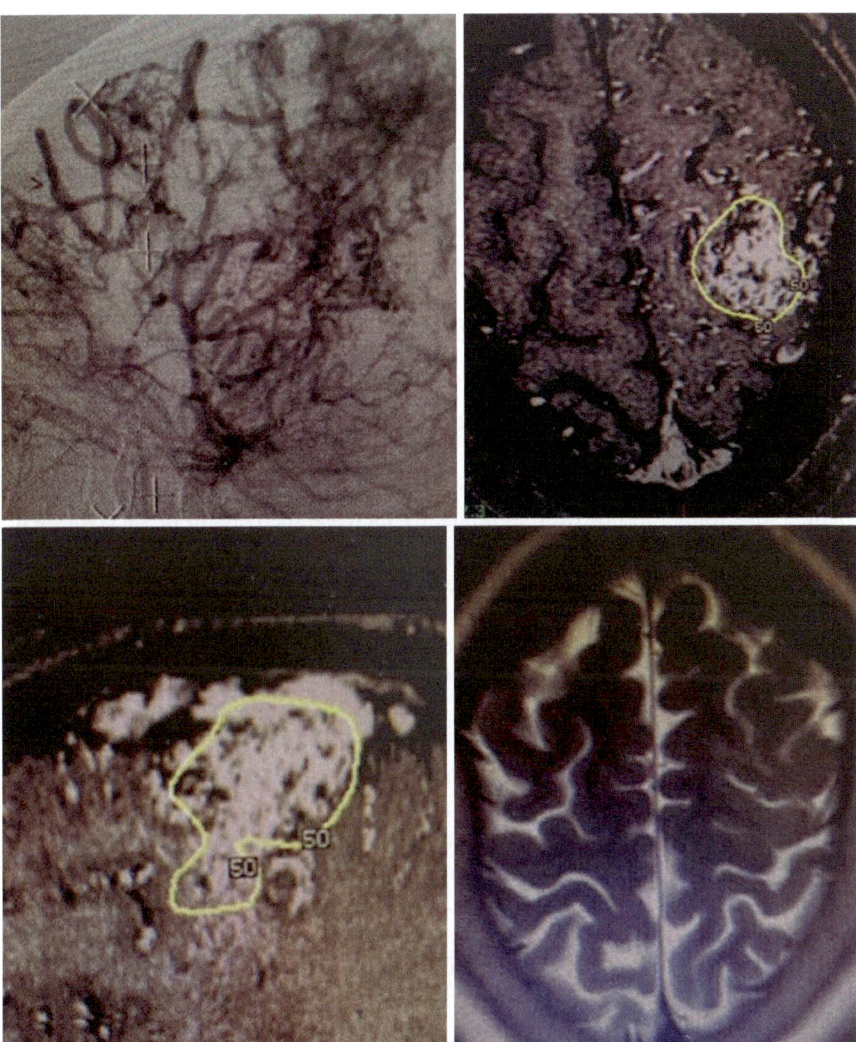

Fig. 5.4 This is a 13-year-old girl who was experiencing right arm and leg tingling episodes and headaches, found to have a moderate sized left frontal AVM with partial moyamoya disease (**a**: the AVM and moyamoya on lateral left carotid angiogram). Gamma Knife was performed (**b**: axial postcontrast T1 MRI from date of treatments; **c**: sagittal postcontrast T1 MRI from date of treatment). MRI from 6 years later shows complete resolution of the AVM (**d**: axial postcontrast T1 weighted MRI). Her symptoms have all resolved

Stroke

Stroke, with Large Vessel Occlusion

There is good evidence that viable patients with acute large vessel occlusions will, on average, benefit from prompt endovascular thrombectomy [29, 30].

Middle Cerebral Artery (MCA) Stroke

Numerous studies—The DESTINY trial [31], the DECIMAL trial [32], the HAMLET trial [33–35], the HeADFIRST trial [36], the DESTINY 2 trial [37], the HeMMI trial [38]—all showed no significant increase in the percent of patients who survived with good functional outcomes after hemicraniectomy for MCA stroke (hemicraniectomy did however significantly increase the percent of survivors with poor functional outcomes). Hemicraniectomy patients who survived were about five times more likely to have a lifelong dependence on others for care (Modified Rankin Scale/MRS 3, 4, or 5) than they were to be functionally independent (MRS 2). No patients survived with an MRS of 0 or 1.

While aggregating data from some of these studies suggested the possibility of a benefit, meta-analysis data found the quality of evidence that hemicraniectomy improved the likelihood of a good functional outcome in patients with MCA strokes to be "low" [39]. Even this conclusion required consideration of (1) studies that themselves showed no benefit; (2) studies that were stopped early; (3) studies that had very different inclusion requirements and different treatment methods; (4) studies that lumped together dominant and non-dominant MCA strokes, partial and complete distribution MCA strokes, and MCA strokes that were isolated as well as MCA strokes concurrent with strokes in other vascular distributions; (5) studies that included patients with significant disability who required lifelong assistance (MRS 3 and 4) as "good functional outcomes." Of interest, the DESTINY 2 trial, of patients over 60 treated with or without hemicraniectomy after a moderate to large MCA stroke, found that not one patient survived who was functionally independent (MRS 0, 1, or 2), and 80% of surviving patients, both surgically and medically managed, subsequently suffered from severe depression.

Nonetheless, there may be some very select group of young healthy patients who suffer acute moderate to large right-sided (non-dominant hemisphere) MCA strokes, and who would otherwise herniate, who may benefit from hemicraniectomy, if the patient (or family) is willing to accept that moderate to severe disability is a much more likely outcome than functional independence. This may be one of the few reasons to even consider a hemicraniectomy. Craniectomy in these cases, for optimum decompression, should be large, and the dura should be widely opened (but can then be covered with a large piece of allograft dura). As benefit is very uncertain for surgery even for an isolated right-sided MCA stroke, there would seem to be little justification for such surgery in the face of a left MCA stroke or an MCA stroke with concurrent strokes in other distributions, as survivors will be left with significant disability. A study that looked at hemicraniectomy for otherwise healthy patients under 60 with isolated right MCA strokes would not be unreasonable.

Cerebellar Stroke

Patients with large cerebellar stroke have a much poorer outcome if there is concurrent infarct of the brainstem or contralateral cerebellum. For large unilateral cerebellar stroke in otherwise viable patients, treatment of hydrocephalus with a ventriculostomy significantly increases the percent of patients with good functional outcomes. Performance of suboccipital craniectomy—whether with duraplasty, removal of infarcted cerebellum, or with ventriculostomy—does not clearly increase the percent of patients who survive with good functional outcomes compared with ventriculostomy alone [40–42]. That being said, there may be a select subgroup of younger, healthier, otherwise viable patients with large unilateral cerebellar strokes (in the absence of brainstem stroke or contralateral cerebellar stroke) who may benefit from suboccipital decompression in addition to ventriculostomy, and this would be worth further investigation.

Chapter 6
Brain Trauma

Traumatic Bleeds/Contusions

As with other intracerebral hemorrhages, there is little evidence that removing traumatic intracerebral bleeds leads to a significant increase in the likelihood of a good recovery. See the earlier section for traumatic epidural hematomas, subdural hematomas, and intraventricular hemorrhages.

Penetrating Brain Injuries

These can usually be irrigated out in the emergency room with just a scalp closure and a brief course of antibiotics. If there remains an object that is penetrating the brain, then removal of the object in the operating room is appropriate.

Skull Fractures

Most of these require no surgery. Linear skull fractures can be left alone. Mild depressed skull fractures that are "closed" (no open laceration over the fracture) can usually be left alone. Mild depressed skull fractures that are "open" (the scalp is lacerated over the fracture) can usually just be washed out and closed in the emergency room. Surgery is appropriate for skull fractures that are significantly depressed [43].

M. H. Brisman, *Put Down the Knife*,
https://doi.org/10.1007/978-3-031-48499-5_6

Intracranial Pressure Monitors/"Bolts"

These are intracranial pressure (ICP) monitors that are usually placed in the right frontal lobe in patients with severe traumatic brain injury—a Glasgow Coma Scale (GCS) of 3–8. The device itself has no therapeutic purpose, and even the information it conveys is not clearly any more useful than close clinical observation in an ICU with frequent serial head CT's. Furthermore, presumably whether there is an ICP monitor recording a high ICP or there is no such monitor, such patients would still be managed with standard measures to minimize intracranial hypertension.

Several large studies [44, 45] showed that the use of intracranial pressure monitors in patients with severe brain injury did not improve the percent of patients who survived with good outcomes. A subsequent randomized controlled study was created, the BEST TRIP trial [46], funded by the NIH, of 324 patients to help further resolve the matter. This study yet again showed no benefit to ICP monitors in head trauma patients. Some doctors dismissed this study because it was performed in South America, suggesting some kind of inferiority of technique or medical care. Of note, the percentage of patients with good outcomes in this study were very similar to those reported in large recent multi-institutional studies such as the CENTER-TBI study [47]. A recent study of children with severe head injury also showed no increase in the likelihood of good outcomes with the use of ICP monitors [48].

As such, many large studies are clear that these devices do not lead to a greater chance of a good clinical outcome, though in combination with other aggressive treatments, they do lead to lower hospital mortality and a greater number of survivors with a poor functional outcome. Their use probably does lead to a greater use of craniectomy, which itself has no demonstrated role in improving good outcomes in trauma patients. ICP monitors do however carry real risk of bleeding, infection, or seizure. As such, while many United States trauma programs currently require placement of these devices, with time, this practice will likely decrease.

Craniectomy for Trauma

Brain trauma is one of the most common settings for the performance of decompressive craniectomy, for issues that may include a high monitored ICP, a generalized brain edema, or a deteriorating clinical picture. Nonetheless, numerous studies—including the DECRA trial [49] and the Rescue ICP trial [50]—have demonstrated that craniectomies do not improve the likelihood of a good clinical outcome in trauma patients. As such, they should rarely be performed for this indication.

Chapter 7
Brain Tumors

Pituitary Tumors

While these are usually spontaneously occurring, isolated tumors, pituitary adenomas can occur as part of multiple endocrine neoplasia type 1 (MEN 1). Pituitary tumors are almost all benign, with only the very rare presentation of a malignant pituitary carcinoma. Pituitary tumors are categorized by size as microadenomas (under 1 cm), macroadenomas (over 1 cm), and giant adenomas (over 4 cm), and as either "secretory" or "non-secretory" depending on whether the tumor produces an excess of a hormone.

Non-secretory

The major concern for these tumors is that they will grow upward and press on the optic nerves/chiasm and cause vision problems (such as a bitemporal hemianopsia). Usually these are only treated if they are at least 1 cm in size. Initial treatment may be endonasal transsphenoidal surgery or stereotactic radiosurgery, depending on the size of the tumor and the degree of chiasmal compression, and the symptoms. The open surgery is usually now performed with an endonasal endoscopic transsphenoidal approach with an ENT surgeon, as this is the least invasive surgical approach (see Fig. 7.1). In removing these pituitary tumors, 3 and 5 mm ring curettes are used to gently remove whatever tumor will come out easily. Complete tumor removal is not necessary for a successful outcome. It is well worthwhile to avoid causing a CSF leak at surgery. If CSF is seen, a repair of some sort must be performed. Placement of a lumbar drain at the time of surgery is helpful in repairing these CSF leaks. Such drains need only be left in for 2–3 days. Patients can usually be sent home after transsphenoidal surgery the following day, with a prescription for DDAVP in case

M. H. Brisman, *Put Down the Knife*,
https://doi.org/10.1007/978-3-031-48499-5_7

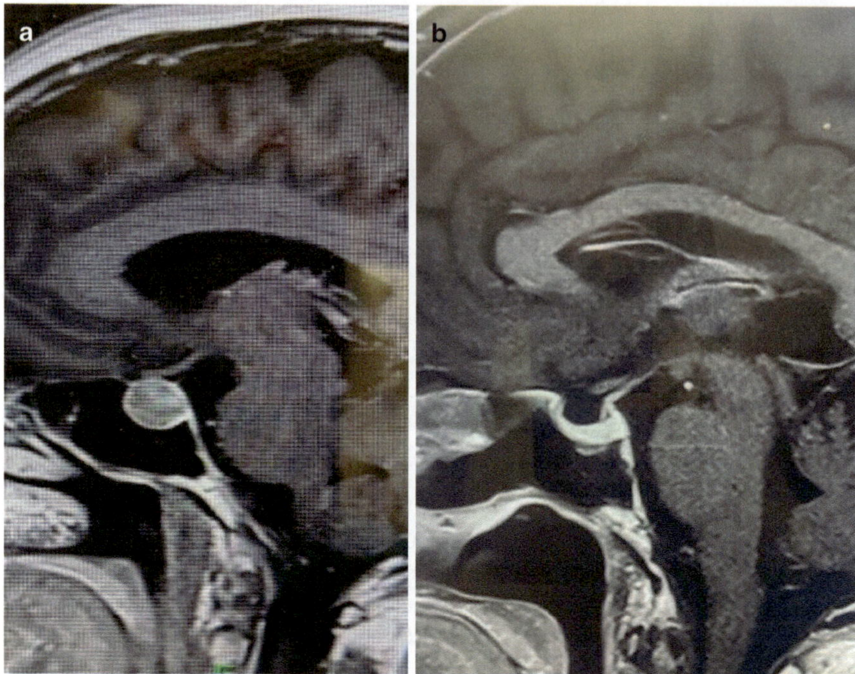

Fig. 7.1 This is a 53-year-old man with several months of persistent bothersome midline frontal headaches. Imaging was consistent with a pituitary macroadenoma just touching the optic nerves (**a**: postcontrast T1 sagittal MRI image). Endocrine testing was normal. The patient underwent endonasal endoscopic transsphenoidal removal of the tumor. Postoperative imaging showed a good removal of the tumor (**b**: postcontrast T1 sagittal MRI image). After surgery, the patient's headaches immediately and completely resolved

their urine output subsequently picks up. Gentle surgical maneuvering usually avoids CSF leaks and postoperative hypopituitarism.

Any significant residual or recurrent tumor can usually be treated with radiosurgery [51] (see Fig. 7.2). As such, repeat surgery for removal of a pituitary tumor is rarely necessary. A tumor that is not compressing the chiasm can usually be treated with radiosurgery [52].

For larger tumors, residual or recurrent, or tumors with some chiasmal compression, hypofractionated radiosurgery in five sessions can be performed (see Fig. 7.3). Standard fractionated radiation therapy can also sometimes be considered.

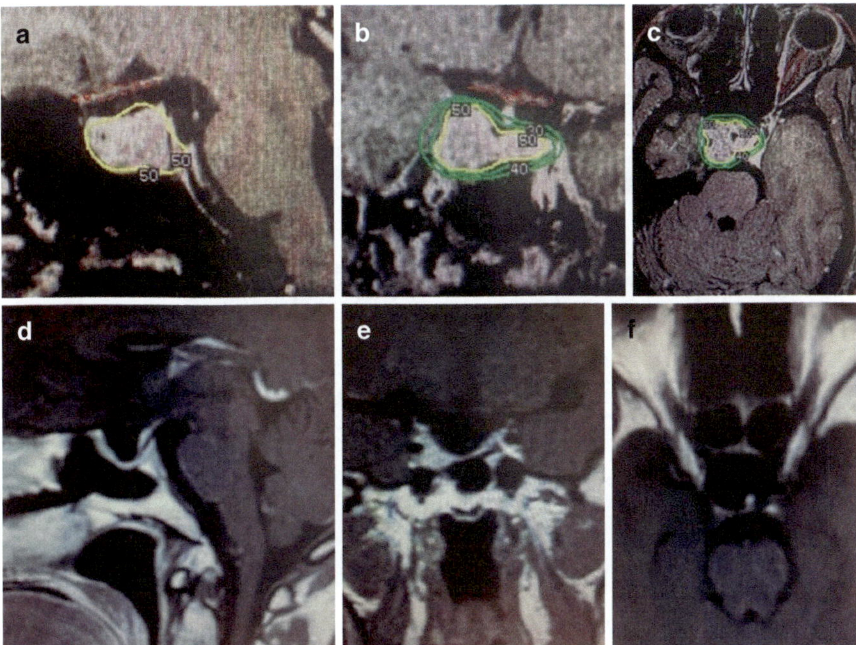

Fig. 7.2 This is a 45-year-old man who 3 years earlier had undergone endoscopic transsphenoidal removal of a non-secretory pituitary macroadenoma. The tumor had now recurred. Gamma Knife was performed (**a**: sagittal T1 postcontrast MRI at the time of Gamma Knife treatment; **b**: coronal T1 postcontrast MRI at the time of Gamma Knife treatment; **c**: axial postcontrast MRI at the time of Gamma Knife treatment). Six years later, the patient remained neurologically intact and takes Synthroid but otherwise has normal pituitary function. MRI shows the tumor has almost completely disappeared (**d**: sagittal T1 postcontrast MRI; **e**: coronal T1 postcontrast MRI; **f**: axial T1 postcontrast MRI)

Secretory

Prolactinomas

These tumors (prolactin secreting) rarely need surgery or radiosurgery and can almost always be managed with just medicines (dopamine agonists), such as cabergoline. Even large tumors causing chiasmal compression and visual disturbances can usually be treated with medication only, which usually yields rapid improvement in symptoms, as well as shrinkage of the tumor and normalization of the prolactin levels (see Figs. 7.4 and 7.5).

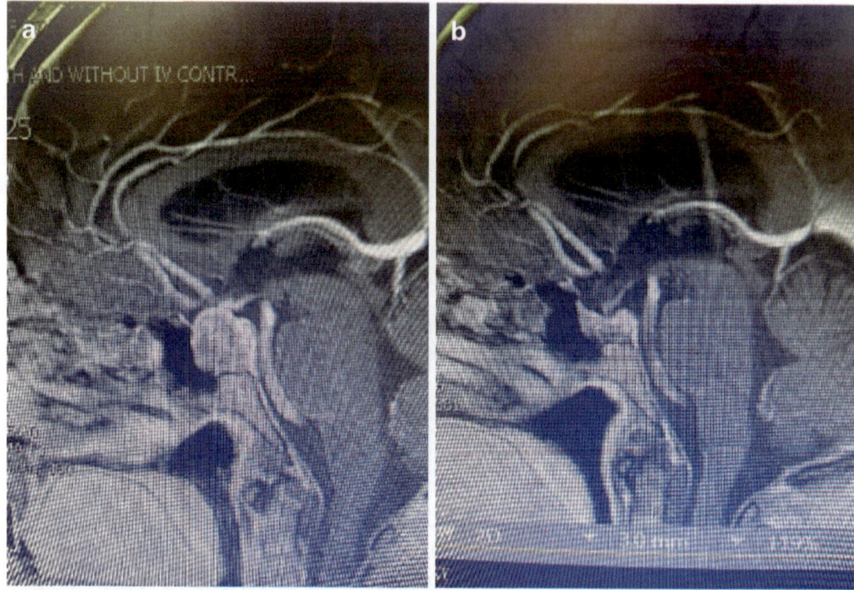

Fig. 7.3 This is a 77-year-old woman who was incidentally found to have a non-secretory macroadenoma that had been enlarging (**a**). Her vision was normal. The tumor came up to the optic chiasm but was not compressing it. She was otherwise healthy. She underwent a five-session hypofractionated radiosurgery treatment. Six years later, the tumor was mostly gone (**b**). The patient was neurologically intact, though she did now take synthroid and hydrocortisone

Cushing's Disease

These tumors (adrenocorticotropic hormone secreting) are usually first managed with attempted removal with an endoscopic transsphenoidal approach. If cortisol levels remain high, radiosurgery can be performed for the remaining tumor, and medicines can also be used (see Fig. 7.6).

Acromegaly/Gigantism

These tumors (growth hormone secreting) are usually first managed with attempted removal with an endoscopic transsphenoidal approach. If IGF-1 levels remain high, radiosurgery can be performed for the remaining tumor, and medicines can also be used. Higher radiosurgery doses are required for secretory tumors than for non-secretory tumors.

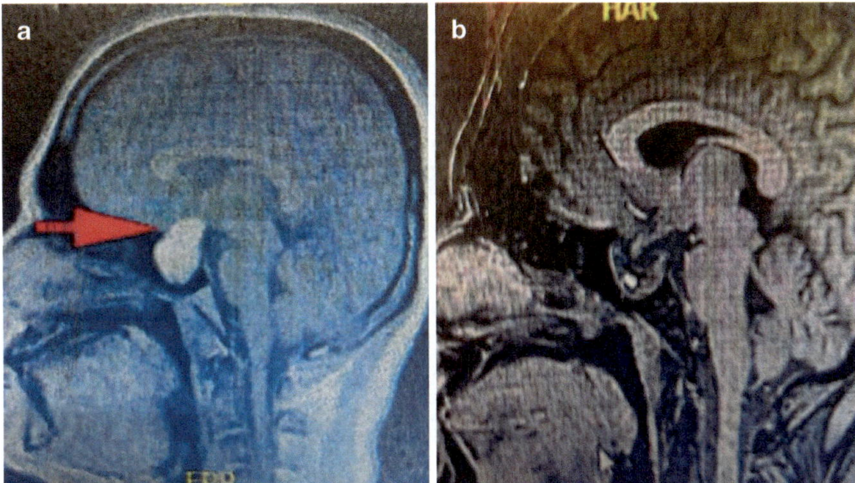

Fig. 7.4 This is a 23-year-old who reported 3 months of significantly blurry vision. He otherwise had no complaints. He felt his vision was not clearly worse than it had been 3 months earlier. Formal ophthalmological testing showed a significant bitemporal hemianopsia. Endocrine tests were all normal except for a prolactin level of 260 ng/mL. MRI showed a 2.8 cm pituitary mass compressing the optic chiasm with slight extension into the left cavernous sinus and a cystic component of indeterminate nature (**a**: sagittal postcontrast). The patient was started on oral cabergoline twice a week. Soon after starting the medicine, he noted his vision was starting to improve. At 4 months follow-up, the patient reported his vision had returned to normal. MRI showed the tumor was no longer visible (**b**: sagittal postcontrast MRI)

Pituitary Apoplexy

When patients present acutely, due to bleed or infarct within a pituitary tumor—and such presentation usually includes an acute bad headache—surgery is generally performed if the patient is having rapid loss of vision [53]. Ophthalmoparesis may also be present, but this, in itself, does not necessarily require emergency surgery. These patients may also have hypopituitarism that will require medical supplementation, such as steroids. If the patient does not need urgent decompressive surgery, these tumors, after apoplexy, sometimes disappear. Follow-up imaging is needed either way.

Lymphocytic Hypophysitis

One mimic of pituitary tumors should be mentioned here. These patients have MRIs that seem to demonstrate a pituitary tumor. The reasons one should suspect the diagnosis of lymphocytic hypophysitis are (1) if the patient is in the later part of a

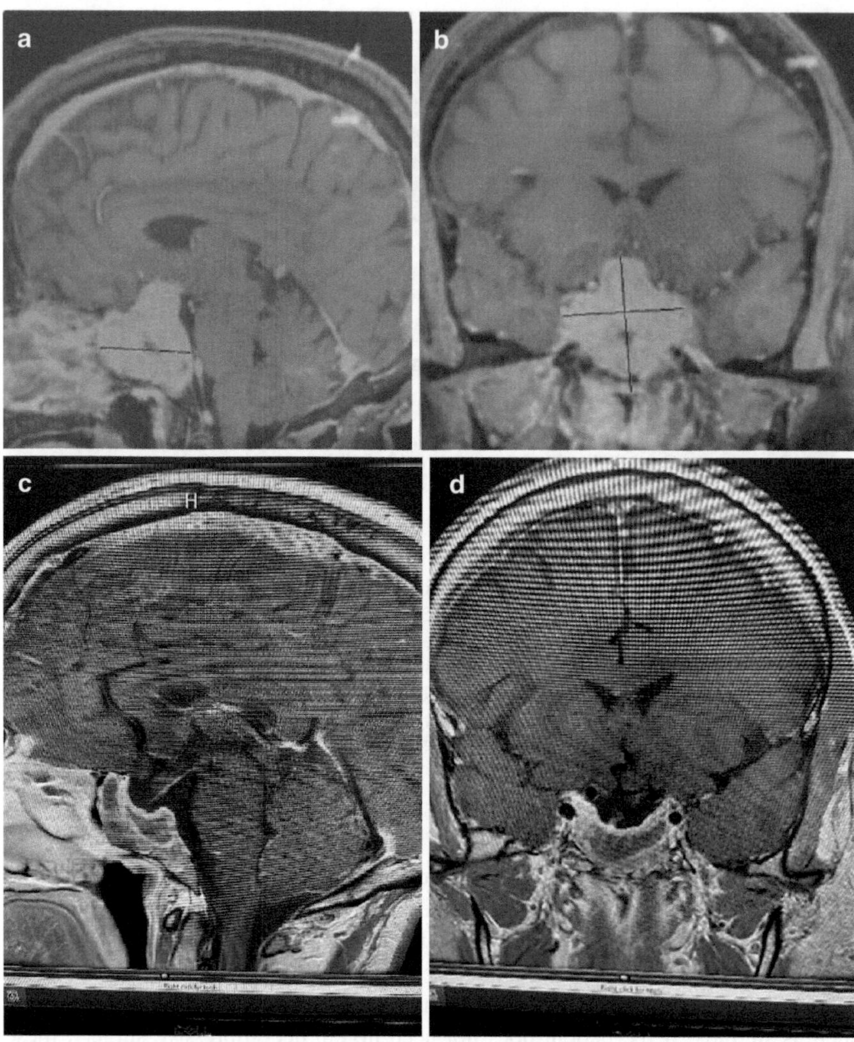

Fig. 7.5 This is a 52-year-old man with several months of progressive headaches and visual loss. Imaging showed a large pituitary region mass (**a**: postcontrast T1 sagittal MRI image; **b**: postcontrast T1 coronal MRI image). His endocrine tests were normal except for a prolactin level of 8000 ng/mL. He was started on oral cabergoline twice a week. Soon thereafter, his headaches had resolved, and his vision had returned to normal. MRI several weeks later showed dramatic reduction in the size of the tumor (**c**: postcontrast T1 sagittal MRI image; **d**: postcontrast T1 coronal MRI image)

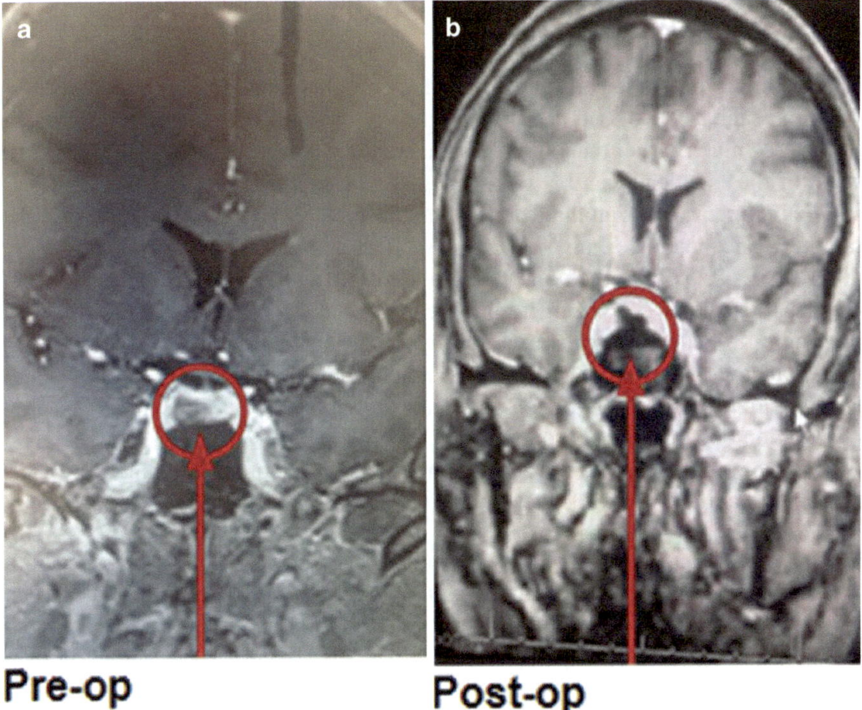

Fig. 7.6 This is a 46-year-old woman who had diabetes, hypertension, and progressive swelling of her face and body, and endocrine testing consistent with Cushing's disease. MRI demonstrated a 9 mm right-sided pituitary adenoma (**a**: postcontrast T1 weighted coronal image). She underwent endonasal endoscopic transsphenoidal removal of the tumor. Postoperative imaging showed the tumor was completely removed (**b**: post-operative postcontrast coronal MRI image). Postoperative lab tests showed very low serum cortisol levels, consistent with a successful operation. She was placed on replacement hydrocortisone which was eventually weaned off. She felt much better, and her diabetes and hypertension were much improved. Her subsequent endocrine testing was consistent with a cure from her Cushing's disease

pregnancy or has recently given birth and (2) if there is a panhypopituitarism that one usually only sees in pituitary tumors that undergo apoplexy. MRI involvement of the pituitary stalk is also suspicious for this disorder. These masses, which represent just enlarged inflamed pituitary tissue, can be mostly managed with a course of steroids [54].

Acoustic Neuromas (Vestibular Schwannomas)

These benign tumors usually present with symptoms related to eighth nerve dysfunction, such as decreased hearing, tinnitus, or dizziness. These tumors are being discovered much earlier than in the past due to the widespread availability of MRIs. Most of these patients can be well-managed with radiosurgery. For most cases, a single treatment with Gamma Knife, with a dose of 12–13 Gy to the margin of the tumor, is adequate (see Figs. 7.7 and 7.8). If the patient has serviceable hearing, doses of 12–12.5 Gy to the tumor margin are used, and it is best to keep the mean cochlear dose below 3 Gy. Larger tumors can often also be treated with radiosurgery but might do better with a five session hypofractionated treatment (or sometimes with standard fractionated radiation treatment). For patients with tumors under 5 mm, patients with stable tumors, and patients who are elderly or in poor health, observation only may be appropriate.

It is the rare patient with an acoustic neuroma who requires a craniotomy. This seems most appropriate when the tumor is very large, maybe over 3.5 × 3.5 × 3.5 cm. In these cases, the tumor can be debulked, without dissecting the tumor off the cranial nerves or drilling the canal, and the remainder of the tumor can be treated with radiosurgery (see Fig. 7.9). Again, this should be a very small number of overall patients seen.

Surgery clearly carries a much higher risk than radiosurgery, with no clear improvement in outcomes, certainly for tumors under 2.5 cm [55]. To the contrary, surgery carries much higher rates of hearing loss, as well as facial weakness, stroke, meningitis, and death, which almost never happen with radiosurgery. And while there may be some miniscule risk of secondary malignancy with stereotactic radiosurgery, that risk is much lower than the approximately 1% risk of death or major morbidity from the open surgery.

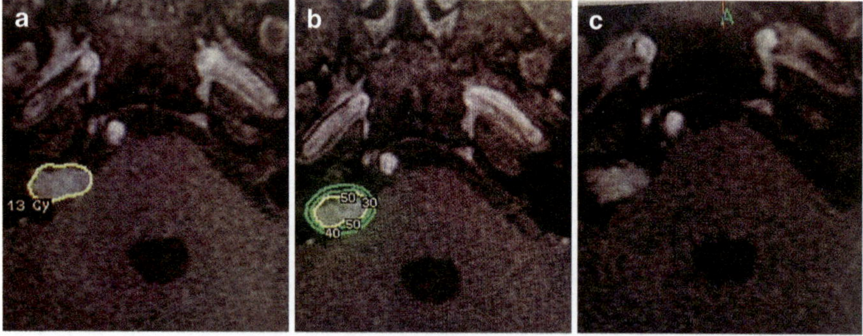

Fig. 7.7 This is a 58-year-old woman found to have decreased hearing in the right ear (about 30% of normal). MRI showed a small right acoustic neuroma. A Gamma Knife treatment was performed (**a**, **b**: axial postcontrast MRI on day of Gamma Knife treatment). 15 years later, her hearing has been preserved at the pre-treatment level and the tumor remains stable on MRI (**c**: T1 axial postcontrast MRI)

Furthermore, data on the complications of acoustic neuroma surgery always significantly understate what surgeons see in actual practice. Surgical patients will often lose hearing, develop facial weakness, develop new dizziness and balance issues, develop chronic headaches, develop facial numbness or pain syndromes, and so on. The risk of both major and minor complications is simply much higher than with radiosurgery.

Gamma Knife is also very safe and effective for younger patients and for patients with neurofibromatosis type 2 (NF-2) who have bilateral acoustic neuromas, though both tumors should not be treated at the same time (see Fig. 7.10). Gamma Knife can also be repeated in the event the tumor keeps growing (about a 5% chance).

I have personally treated about 200 patients with acoustic neuromas and have no patients who have died or developed any permanent facial weakness (and just a handful with transient facial palsy). When I choose to treat someone with a procedure, I usually use Gamma Knife, and for large tumors that I think need surgery, I just debulk the tumor and use radiosurgery for the remainder.

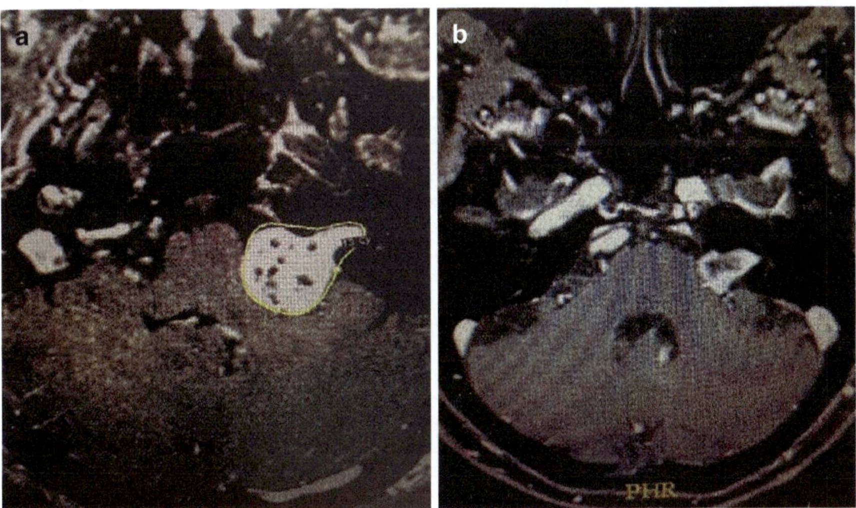

Fig. 7.8 This is a 66-year-old woman who presented with decreased hearing in the left ear and was found to have a 2.3 cm left acoustic neuroma indenting the brainstem. She underwent Gamma Knife treatment (**a**: postcontrast T1 weighted axial MRI image from the day of Gamma Knife treatment). Six years later, she still has hearing in the left ear, though it is less than when the tumor was first treated. MRI shows a dramatic reduction in the size of the tumor (**b**: postcontrast T1 axial MRI)

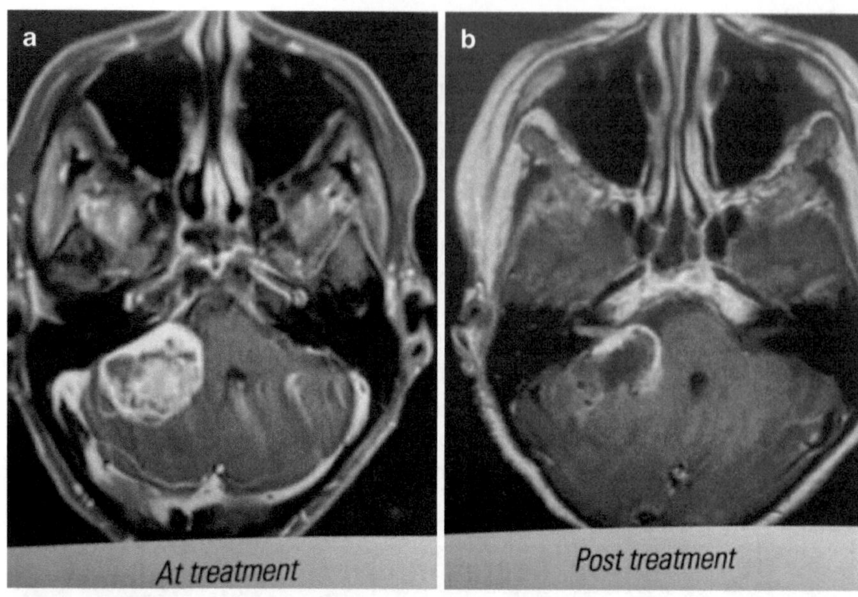

Fig. 7.9 This is a 70-year-old woman who had a large acoustic neuroma that had been enlarging fairly rapidly, who presented now with balance problems and serviceable hearing (**a**: postcontrast axial T1 weighted MRI image). She underwent a retrosigmoid suboccipital craniectomy and debulking of the tumor. Postoperatively, her balance was improved, and her hearing remained unchanged. MRI showed most of the tumor had been removed (**b**: postcontrast axial T1 weighted MRI image). She subsequently underwent radiosurgery treatment for the small remaining piece of tumor

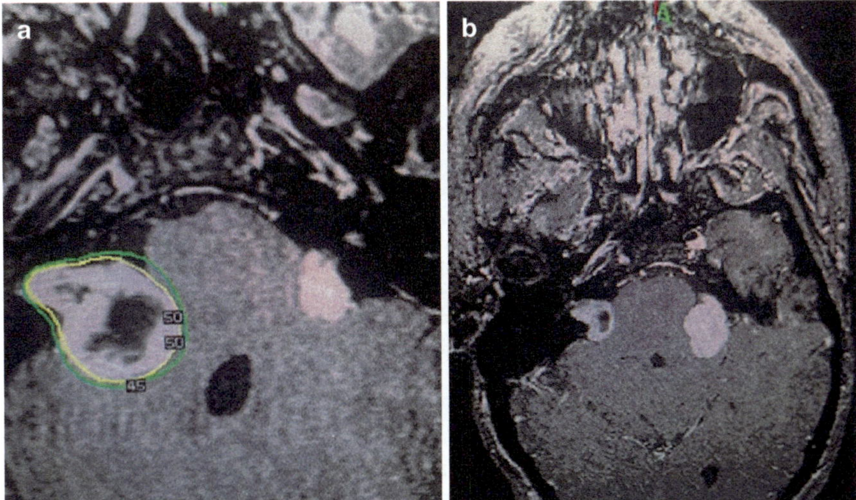

Fig. 7.10 This is a 26-year-old woman with neurofibromatosis type 2 (NF-2) who presented with significant decreased hearing in the right ear (about 10% of normal). MRI showed a large right acoustic neuroma with brainstem compression, and a much smaller left acoustic neuroma. Gamma Knife was performed on the right acoustic neuroma (**a**: postcontrast T1 weighted axial image from the date of Gamma Knife treatment). Six years later, the hearing in the right ear had improved significantly to about 80% of normal. MRI (**b**: postcontrast T1 weighted axial image) showed significant reduction in the size of the right acoustic neuroma, but some enlargement of the left acoustic neuroma (which was subsequently treated with Gamma Knife as well)

Brain Meningiomas

These tumors, which are almost always benign, can occur almost anywhere within the cranium. They can be single or multiple (meningiomatosis). Usually no definite cause is found, though they can rarely occur in the setting of NF-2, in patients with familial meningiomatosis, or in patients who have received brain radiation many years earlier.

The vast majority of these tumors can be treated either with observation or with radiosurgery/Gamma Knife [56] (see Fig. 7.11). Even somewhat larger tumors can often be treated with radiosurgery, either with 5 dose hypofractionation (see Fig. 7.12) or by staging the treatment in two or more sessions, usually months apart. Sometimes even standard fractionated radiation can be used.

Open craniotomy should be reserved for those very large symptomatic tumors that just cannot be treated with radiosurgery, and this decision is often best deferred to a neurosurgeon who frequently performs both open surgery for meningiomas and stereotactic radiosurgery. Common locations of large meningiomas that can be successfully removed include the convexity (see Fig. 7.13), the falx (see Fig. 7.14), the sphenoid wing (see Fig. 7.15), the tentorium (see Fig. 7.16), the olfactory groove/planum sphenoidale (see Fig. 7.17) region, and the ventricles.

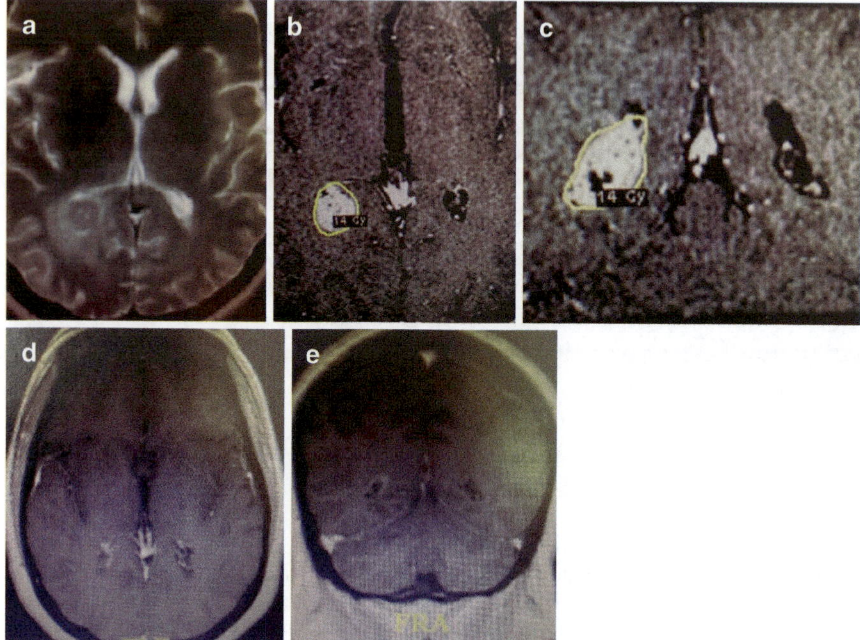

Fig. 7.11 This is a 52-year-old woman who was found incidentally to have a right atrial meningioma with some surrounding edema (**a**: T2 weighted axial MRI image). A Gamma Knife treatment was performed (**b**: postcontrast T1 axial MRI image demonstrating the Gamma Knife treatment plan; **c**: postcontrast T1 coronal MRI image demonstrating the Gamma Knife treatment plan). Three years later, the patient remains without symptoms and the MRI shows the tumor is gone (**d**: postcontrast T1 axial MRI image; **e**: postcontrast T1 coronal image)

Meningiomas usually have well-defined planes between the tumor and normal brain tissue, and often the best way to separate the tumor from the surrounding brain tissue is with the sequential use of multiple surgical cottonoids. Such classic dissection technique is often referred to as a "cottonoid dissection" (see Fig. 7.18).

If surgery is deemed to be necessary, it is prudent here, as in most cases, not to try to dissect the tumor off cranial nerves or vital blood vessels if it is stuck to these structures. It is better to minimize risk and treat any tumor that remains with radiosurgery. For the rare higher grade meningiomas (aggressive grade 2's, or grade 3's/malignant), wide field standard radiation may be an appropriate option.

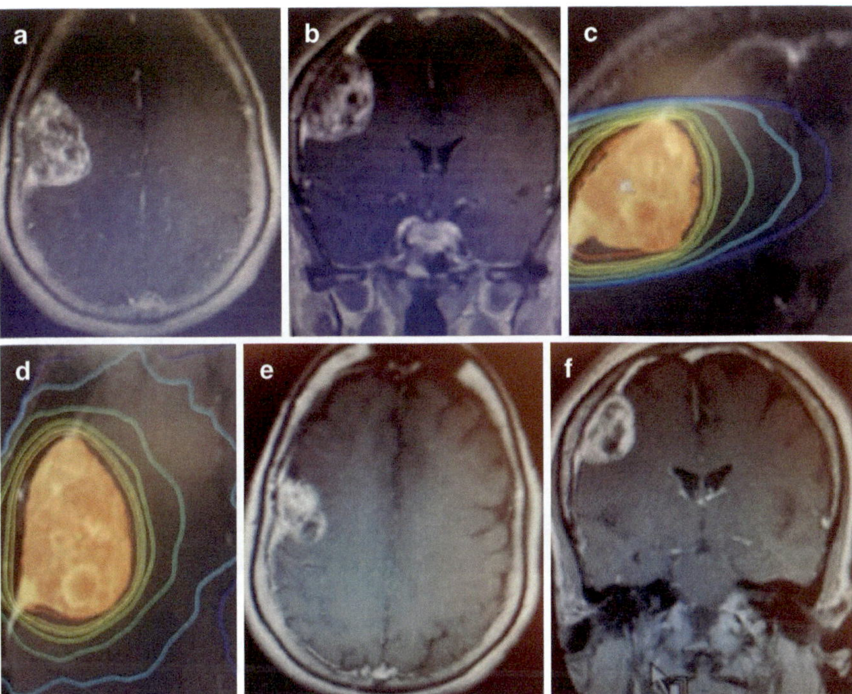

Fig. 7.12 This is a 67-year-old female physician who experienced some intermittent dizziness and was found to have a moderate sized partly cystic meningioma, which had been gradually enlarging over time (**a**: postcontrast T1 axial MRI image; **b**: postcontrast T1 coronal MRI image). She opted for stereotactic radiosurgery treatment. A Novalis radiosurgery treatment was performed over five sessions (**c**: coronal planning images for Novalis treatment; **d**: axial planning images for Novalis treatment). Three years later, the patient had no symptoms, and the tumor was much smaller (**e**: postcontrast T1 axial MRI images; **f**: postcontrast T1 coronal MRI images)

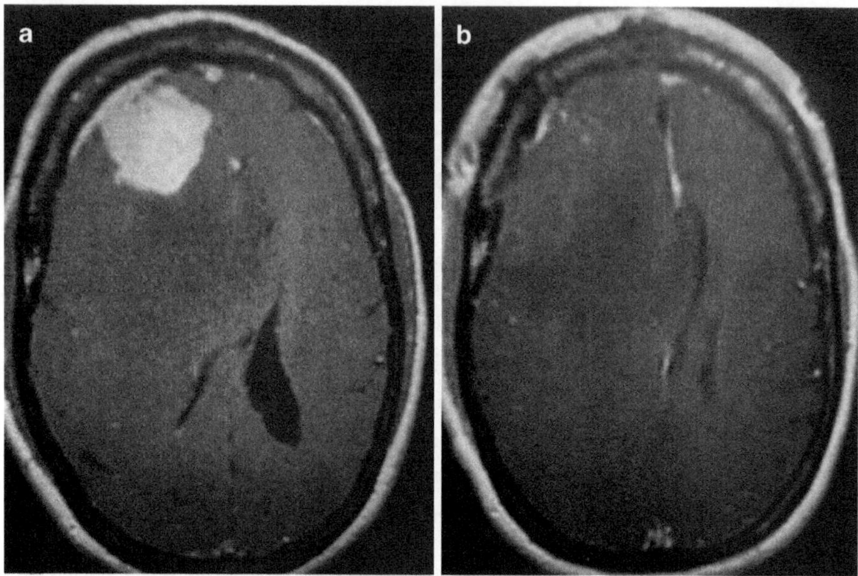

Fig. 7.13 This is a 54-year-old woman with progressive headaches found to have a right frontal convexity meningioma with enormous surrounding edema and midline shift (**a**: postcontrast T1 weighted axial MRI). Her tumor was removed via a right frontal craniotomy. Her pre-operative headaches fully resolved. Post-op images show complete removal of the tumor (**b**: postcontrast T1 weighted axial MRI images)

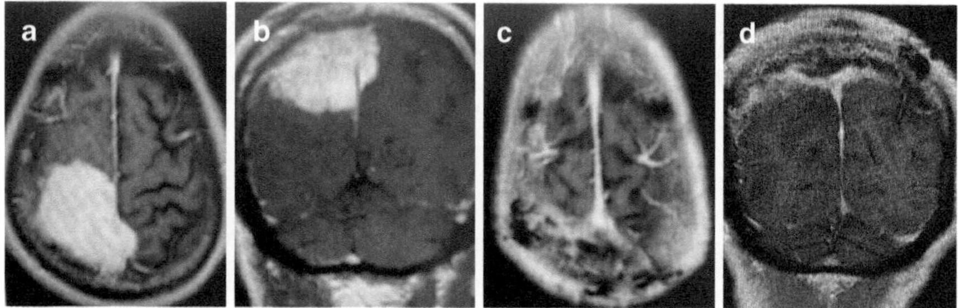

Fig. 7.14 This is a 68-year-old man who was having progressive weakness of his left arm and leg and was found to have a large right parietal meningioma involving the falx and convexity, growing off somewhat to the left side as well and filling a portion of the superior sagittal sinus (**a**: postcontrast T1 axial MRI image; **b**: postcontrast T1 coronal MRI image). The tumor was removed via a bilateral parietal craniotomy with resection of the involved segment of the superior sagittal sinus. His pre-operative symptoms all resolved. His postoperative MRI showed a good removal of the tumor (**c**: postcontrast T1 axial MRI image; **d**: postcontrast coronal T1 MRI image)

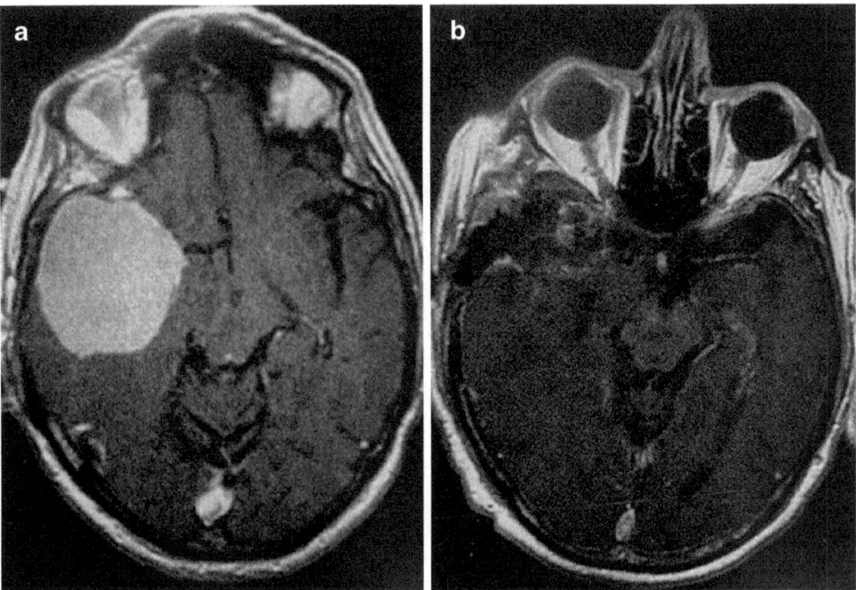

Fig. 7.15 This is an 80-year-old man with personality changes found to have a 6 cm right sphenoid wing/temporal meningioma (**a**: postcontrast axial T1 weighted MRI image). Using a right fronto-temporal craniotomy, the tumor was separated from the sylvian vessels and removed in entirety (**b**: postcontrast T1 weighted axial MRI image). Subsequently, his pre-operative symptoms all resolved

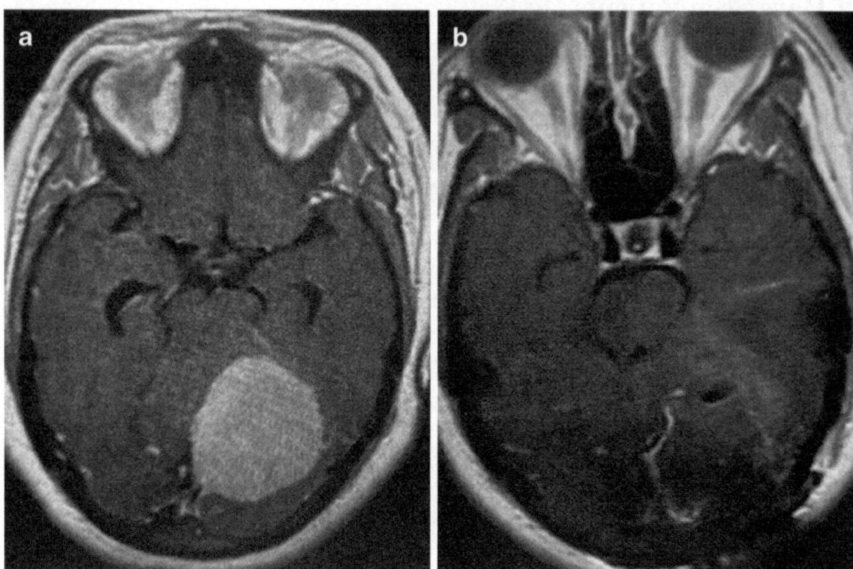

Fig. 7.16 This is a 53-year-old woman who experienced progressive headaches and unsteadiness, found to have a 5 cm left posterior fossa meningioma growing inferiorly from the tentorium with midline shift and early hydrocephalus (**a**: postcontrast T1 weighted axial MRI image). The tumor was removed via a combined left occipital/suboccipital craniectomy with resection of a portion of the left tentorium and subsequent cranioplasty. A temporary right frontal ventriculostomy was placed and later removed. The patient's pre-operative symptoms all subsequently resolved. Postoperative MRI showed good removal of the tumor with less mass effect on the brainstem and normalization of the ventricular size (**b**: postcontrast T1 weighted axial MRI image)

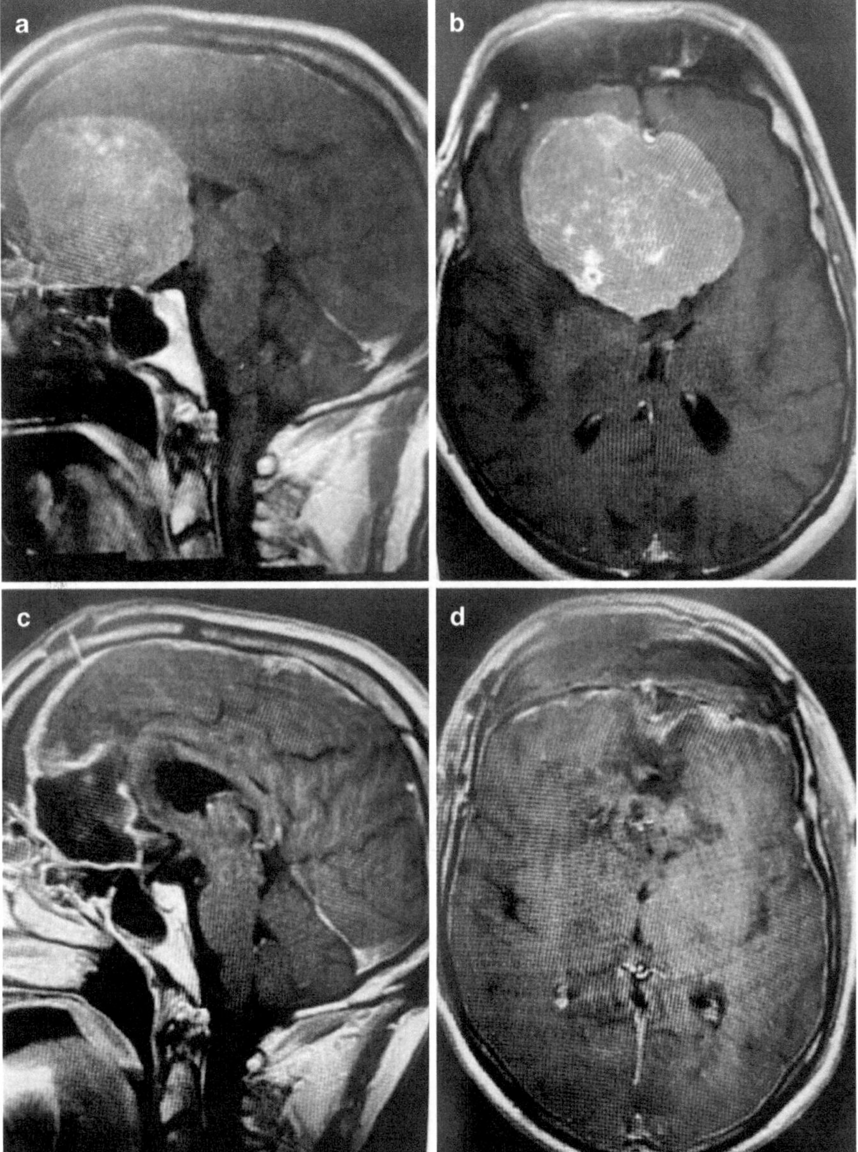

Fig. 7.17 This is a 70-year-old man who presented with gait imbalance and personality changes found to have a 7.5 cm olfactory groove meningioma (**a**: postcontrast T1 sagittal MRI image; **b**: postcontrast T1 axial MRI image). The tumor was removed via a bifrontal craniotomy, subfrontal approach, with exenteration of the frontal sinus. Postoperatively, all pre-operative symptoms resolved. Postoperative MRI showed complete removal of the tumor (**c**: postcontrast T1 sagittal MRI image; **d**: postcontrast T1 axial MRI image)

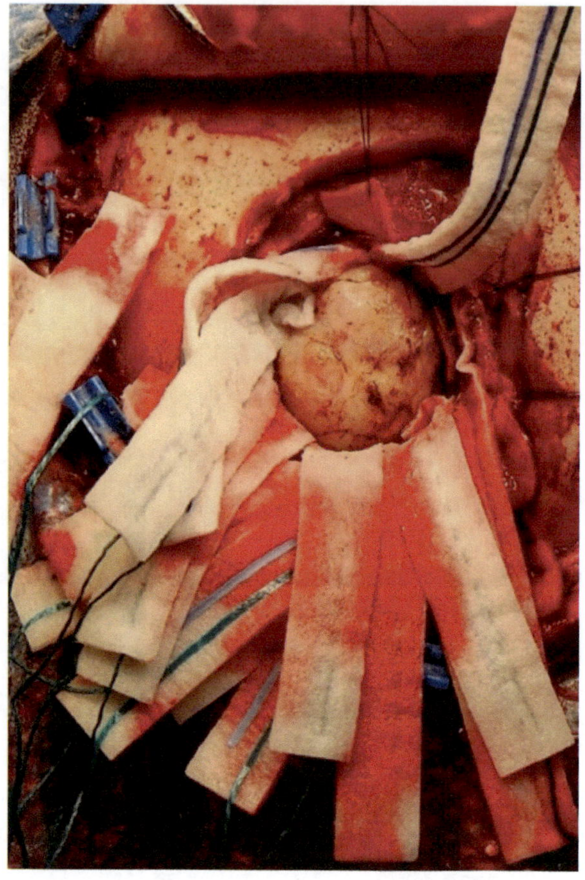

Fig. 7.18 This is an intraoperatvie image showing a left parietal craniotomy and a "cottonoid dissection" to separate a falx meningioma from the surrounding brain tissue

Brain Metastases

These represent the most common malignant brain tumors. Craniotomy is rarely needed in these cases.

For most patients, one day outpatient Gamma Knife treatment will be the best option (see Fig. 7.19). Standard whole brain radiation treatment takes several weeks, causes hair loss and fatigue, and can cause memory loss for longer term survivors. Nonetheless, for some patients with innumerable lesions, or in patients with multiple large metastases, whole brain radiation therapy is perfectly reasonable and appropriate.

Generally, in the case of solitary metastasis, it has been found that craniotomy leads to no better results than Gamma Knife treatment [57], so it is unclear why those patients should be undergoing surgery. Furthermore, the craniotomy patients will still need either follow-up radiosurgery or standard fractionated radiation to minimize recurrences.

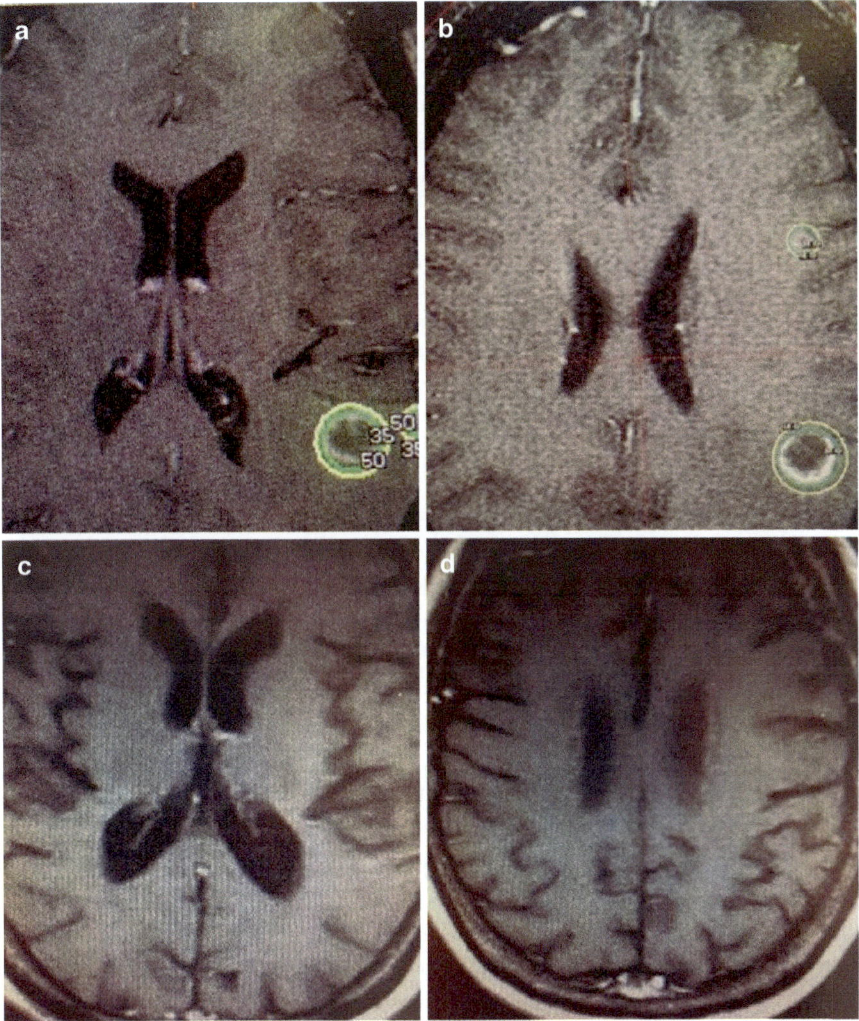

Fig. 7.19 This is a 61-year-old woman with non-small cell lung cancer found to have three brain metastases, one left frontal and two left parietal. A Gamma Knife treatment was performed in which all three tumors were treated at the same time (**a**: postcontrast T1 axial image from the time of Gamma Knife treatment; **b**: postcontrast T1 axial image, more superior, also from the time of Gamma Knife treatment). Six years later, the patient remained neurologically intact, and MRI showed the tumors were all gone (**c**: postcontrast T1 axial MRI image; **d**: postcontrast T1 axial image, more superior cut)

The rare situation in which open surgery might be appropriate would be for a very large metastatic tumor, preferably solitary, that comes close to the surface, in a non-eloquent region, in an otherwise younger and viable patient, with controlled systemic disease. One could also make an argument in a patient who was actively deteriorating due to mass effect from the tumor, despite steroids. When a craniotomy is performed for a brain metastasis, postoperative radiation therapy is necessary for optimal tumor control. In cases of surgery for a single metastasis, radiation or radiosurgery can be limited to the tumor resection area.

Edema around brain metastases is common, including symptomatic edema, but this is not in itself an indication for surgery. Metastatic tumors frequently have edema, which is often readily responsive to dexamethasone treatment. Many surgeons are not aware of how successful radiation can be for most brain metastases. Even patients with multiple large metastases will often show significant tumor reduction and good palliative results with whole brain radiation.

It should also be understood that for most patients with brain metastases, the goal is palliation, not cure. Fortunately, however, there are some patients with brain metastases, who can see a long-term survival. These patients generally have well controlled systemic disease.

Gliomas: Grades 1, 2, 3, 4

Stereotactic neuro-navigation is often quite helpful for those patients who require excision or biopsy of their gliomas. When a diagnostic tissue biopsy is necessary, a stereotactic needle biopsy will usually be adequate (and a craniotomy is rarely necessary).

Grade 1: Juvenile Pilocytic Astrocytoma (JPA)

These are usually discovered during childhood. It is, however, possible, for such a tumor to be found in early adulthood. These are benign tumors. Depending on the location, size, and symptoms, either surgical removal or Gamma Knife radiosurgery may be reasonable treatments. These patients usually do very well, so long as no damage is done during the course of open surgery. Because these tumors are benign, this again argues for not trying to aggressively dissect these tumors off critical brain structures.

Grade 2: Intermediate Grade Gliomas

These tumors have often been called "low-grade gliomas," which is a bit of a misnomer, as these tumors are often fatal and often do not behave like typical benign tumors. For example, these tumors are frequently infiltrative, do not have well-defined borders, and can transform into higher grade gliomas. Intermediate grade gliomas usually present during adulthood. If the tumor is in a non-eloquent region and can be removed in entirety (or at least what is seen on MRI), that would be reasonable [58] (see Figs. 7.20 and 7.21). But that often cannot be done. As such, removing most of the tumor, if that can safely be done, may be best. If the tumor is

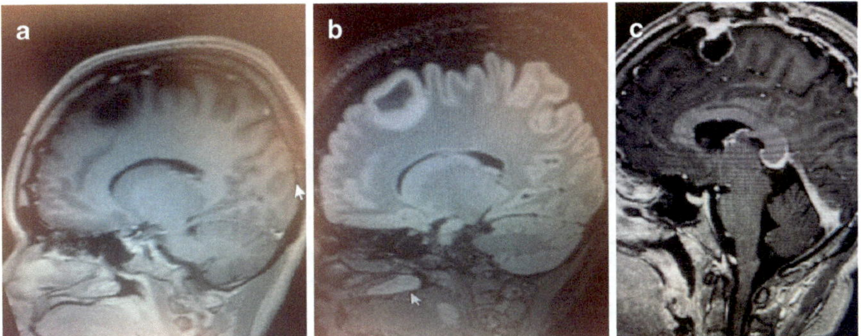

Fig. 7.20 This is a 32-year-old woman who presented with a seizure. She had no further seizures once Keppra was started. Her MRI showed a non-enhancing mass in the left frontal lobe consistent with an intermediate grade glioma (**a**: postcontrast T1 sagittal; **b**: flair sagittal). The tumor was removed via a left frontal craniotomy with neuronavigation assistance. Postoperative images showed a good resection (**c**: postcontrast T1 sagittal). Flair images showed just a small residual. The patient remained neurologically intact. Pathology showed a grade 2 astrocytoma. It was decided to observe the patient with follow-up images

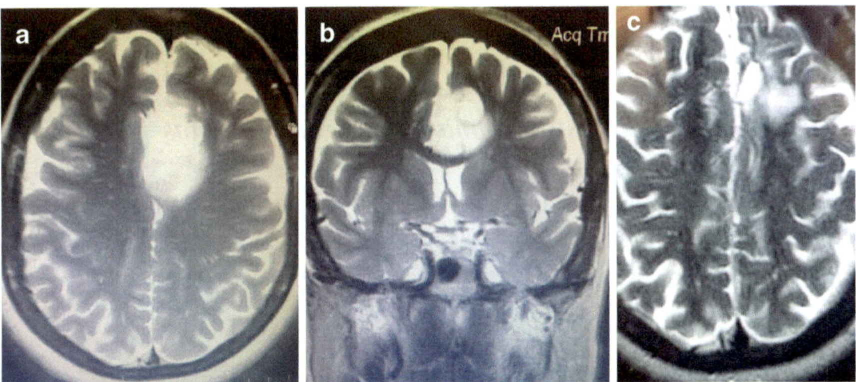

Fig. 7.21 This is a 51-year-old woman with episodes of confusion found on MRI to have a left frontal mass consistent with a glioma. The mass was non-enhancing (**a**: T2 weighted axial MRI image; **b**: T2 weighted coronal MRI image). The episodes of confusion were thought to be seizures and stopped when the patient was started on Keppra. A left frontal craniotomy was performed, and the tumor was removed. Pathology was consistent with an oligodendroglioma. The patient was treated with external beam radiation and temozolomide chemotherapy. Four years later, the patient remained intact and the images were stable (**c**: T2 weighted axial MRI image)

in an eloquent location, a biopsy only may be best. Regardless, surgery can be followed by radiation or chemotherapy depending on the circumstances. Radiosurgery or standard radiation can also be used depending on the circumstance (for example, if there is a recurrent spot of tumor that develops after standard radiation therapy) (see Fig. 7.22). There are likely some intermediate grade gliomas that will do just as well with radiation only as with surgery (with or without radiation), and this would be an appropriate topic for further investigation.

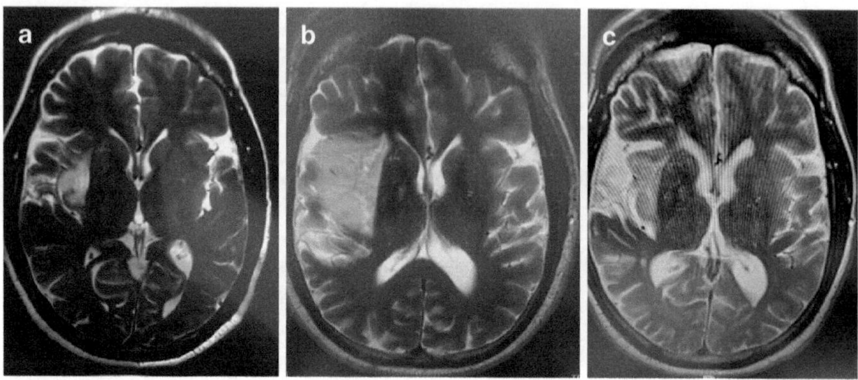

Fig. 7.22 This is a 60-year-old man who was incidentally found to have a small right insular mass felt to be most consistent with an intermediate grade glioma (**a**: T2 weighted axial MRI image). It did not enhance. It was decided to observe this abnormality with follow-up imaging. The patient was then lost to follow-up and returned 9 years later with a complaint of brief episodes of feeling somewhat off and not being able to speak during those episodes. These were thought to be seizures, and the episodes stopped with Keppra. A new MRI was ordered that showed significant enlargement of the mass (**b**: T2 weighted axial MRI). After discussion with the patient, it was decided to treat the patient with external beam radiation treatment. Four years later, the patient remains neurologically intact on the Keppra, and MRI shows dramatic reduction in the size of the insular tumor (**c**: T2 weighted axial MRI image)

Grade 3: Anaplastic Astrocytoma/High Grade Gliomas

The higher grade gliomas tend to develop in older adults. Some of them may have developed initially from intermediate grade gliomas. If a large amount of tumor can be safely removed, this is reasonable. Otherwise, biopsy only may be appropriate, especially in older individuals. Surgery can be followed by radiation, chemotherapy (often temozolomide), and possibly radiosurgery for focal recurrences.

Grade 4: Glioblastoma/High Grade Gliomas

Glioblastoma (GBM) is the most common primary brain malignancy. If most of the enhancing tumor can be safely removed, it is reasonable to do so. Any treatment for such patients must, at this time, be viewed as palliative, due to the poor prognosis that this diagnosis carries even under the best of circumstances. There is clearly a need for better treatments for this disease. Surgical removal of most of the mass, radiation therapy, and chemotherapy (with temozolomide) seem to provide the best current options [59] (see Fig. 7.23). Radiosurgery can be considered for focal recurrences that occur after the initial radiation treatment.

The benefits of repeat operations for gliomas are usually overestimated. For example, a study by Gonzalez et al. [60] showed no benefit to re-operation for glioblastoma. Such surgery usually has much higher rates of complications and much

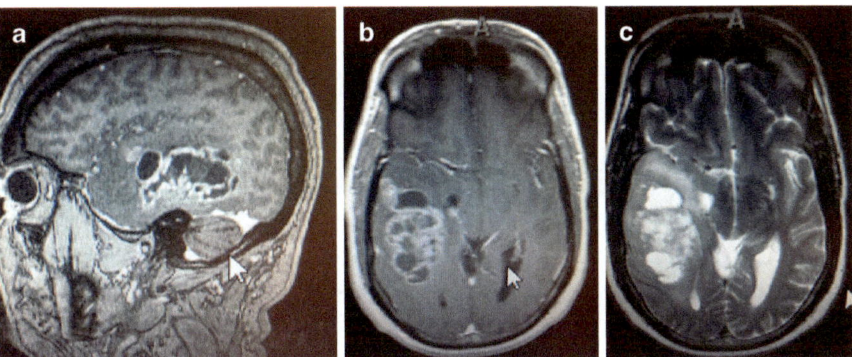

Fig. 7.23 This is a 67-year-old woman who presented with headaches and was found to have a large right posterior temporal mass that enhanced and had both solid and cystic components (**a**: postcontrast T1 sagittal MRI image; **b**: postcontrast T1 axial MRI image; **c**: T2 axial MRI image). The images were felt to be most consistent with a glioblastoma. The patient underwent right temporal craniotomy with stereotactic neuronavigation and debulking of the tumor. Pathology confirmed the diagnosis of glioblastoma. Postoperatively, the patient's headache resolved, and she remained neurologically intact. She was subsequently treated with external beam radiation therapy and temozolomide chemotherapy. One year postoperatively, she had a recurrence of tumor that was treated with stereotactic radiosurgery. The patient succumbed to her disease 2 years and 2 months after her original surgery

less benefit than the original surgery. Patients will usually be at least as well off with radiosurgery, standard radiation, medical management, or no treatment, rather than a repeat brain operation in these cases.

Pineal Tumors

A rare location for a brain tumor in an adult is the pineal region. Tumors in this area can be of many different varieties. The three most common types of tumors in this region are (1) germ cell tumors, (2) pineal gland tumors, and (3) gliomas. Germ cell tumors include germinoma, choriocarcinoma, embryonal carcinoma, endodermal sinus tumor (also known as yolk sac tumor), mixed germ cell tumors, and teratomas (immature teratoma, mature teratoma, and teratoma with malignant transformation). Pineal gland tumors include pineocytoma, pineal parenchymal tumor, papillary pineal tumor, and pineoblastoma.

Work-up can include a spinal MRI series and CSF analysis. Stereotactic biopsy or open surgery may both be appropriate. A biopsy may avoid an extensive craniotomy in the case of pineal germinomas, which are very sensitive to adjuvant therapy. The two traditional surgical approaches to this region are the supracerebellar and the occipital-transtentorial. The occipital-transtentorial approach has the major advantage of avoiding having the patient operated on in the sitting position, which is a challenging position for both the surgeon and the anesthesiologist (see Fig. 7.24). This problem can sometimes be partly mitigated for the supracerebellar approach

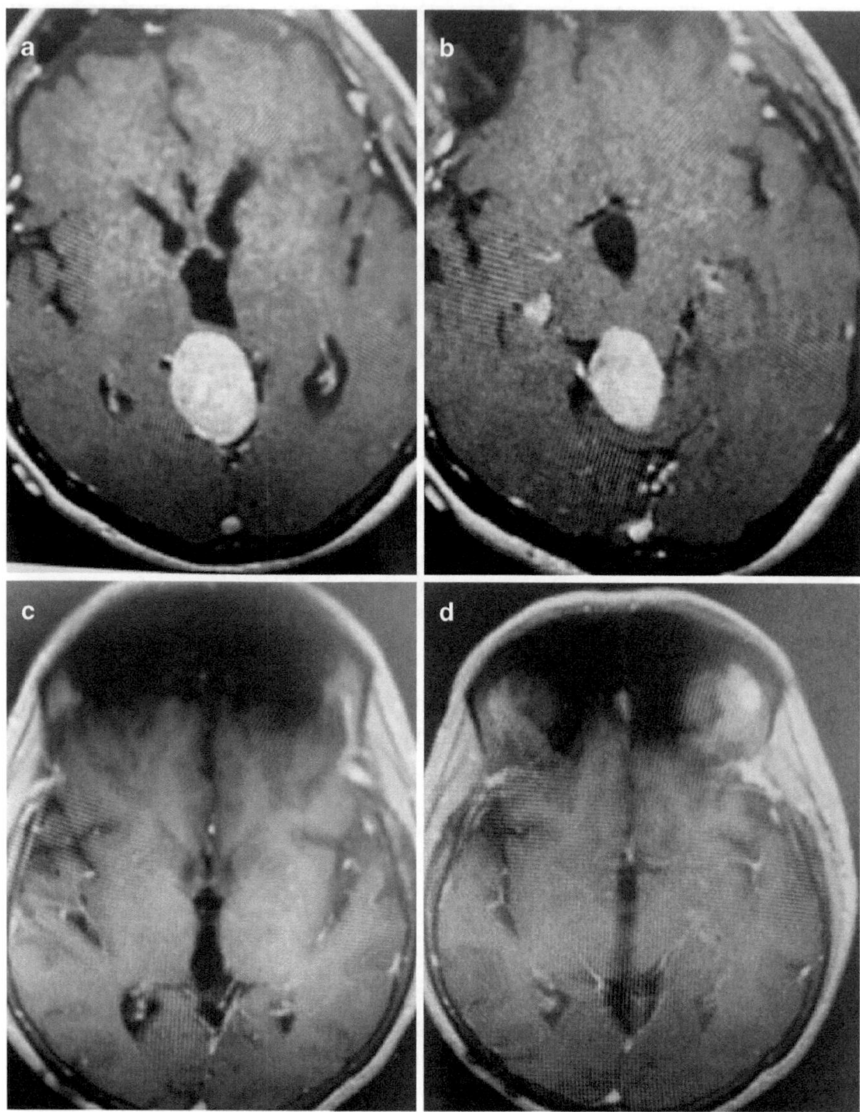

Fig. 7.24 This is a 57-year-old woman with new onset memory problems and gait difficulty found to have a 3 cm pineal region meningioma growing inferiorly off the right tentorium causing compression of the upper brainstem and hydrocephalus (**a**: postcontrast T1 axial MRI image; **b**: postcontrast T1 axial image, a more inferior cut). The tumor was removed via a right occipital/transtentorial approach. Subsequently, the hydrocephalus resolved and did not require shunting. Her pre-operative symptoms all resolved. Follow-up MRI imaging showed the tumor was gone (**c**: postcontrast T1 axial MRI image; **d**: postcontrast T1 axial MRI, a more inferior cut)

by performing the surgery in the lateral position with the head partly tilted up. During pineal tumor surgery, regardless of the approach, the deep cerebral veins must be preserved, as injury to such veins can lead to a disabling deep venous stroke. Tumors in this region may benefit from surgery, standard radiation, radiosurgery, or chemotherapy, depending on the specific circumstances.

Intraventricular Tumors

While many types of brain tumors can secondarily grow into the ventricles, there are a handful of solid brain tumors that generally arise primarily within the ventricular system itself. These tumors can be of different pathological types and can occur in different locations. Intraventricular masses pose unique management issues because they are deep and frequently cause hydrocephalus.

Tumors of the Lateral Ventricle

Neurocytomas are benign tumors that can arise in the lateral ventricles, usually the frontal horn. Subependymal giant cell astrocytomas (SEGA) are benign tumors that arise in the frontal horn around the foramina of Monroe, usually in patients with tuberous sclerosis (one of the phakomatoses/neurocutaneous syndromes). Meningiomas are benign tumors that can rarely occur in the lateral ventricle, including the atrium of the ventricle.

Neurocytomas, subependymal giant cell astrocytomas, and meningiomas in the lateral ventricle that are large may need surgical removal. Such surgery is often best accomplished with the use of a tubular retractor placed under stereotactic neuronavigation guidance (see Figs. 7.25, 7.26, and 7.27). It is critical to take care not to

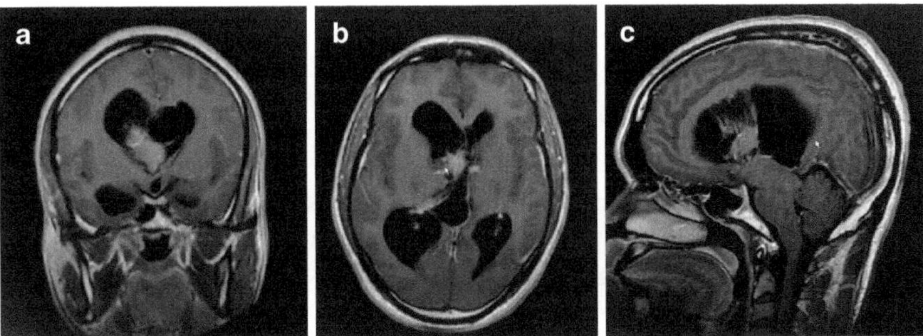

Fig. 7.25 This is a 28-year-old man who presented with recent headaches, memory problems, and urinary incontinence found to have a large mass in the right lateral ventricle extending into the third ventricle through the foramen of Monroe (**a**: postcontrast T1 coronal MRI image; **b**: postcontrast T1 axial MRI image; **c**: postcontrast sagittal image). The tumor was removed via a right frontal craniotomy, with a transcortical approach using a tubular retractor and the operating microscope. Postoperatively, the patient made a full neurological recovery, but did require placement of a ventriculoperitoneal shunt. Pathology showed a neurocytoma. Three years later, a small local recurrence was treated with Gamma Knife

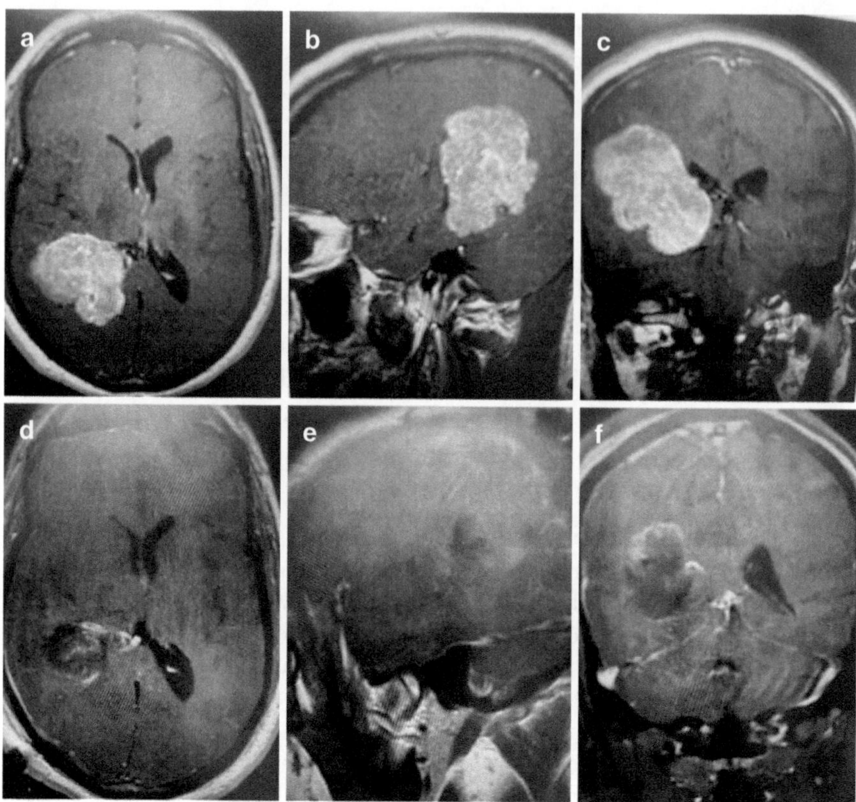

Fig. 7.26 This is a 45-year-old man with headaches, nausea, and blurry vision, found to have a large meningioma arising from the atrium of the right lateral ventricle (**a**: postcontrast T1 weighted axial MRI; **b**: postcontrast T1 weighted sagittal MRI; **c**: postcontrast T1 weighted coronal MRI). His tumor was removed via a right parietal craniotomy and transcortical approach through the superior parietal lobule using the Vycor tubular retractor and the operating microscope. Postoperatively, his symptoms all resolved. Postoperative images showed the tumor was successfully removed (**d**: postcontrast T1 weighted axial MRI image; **e**: postcontrast T1 weighted sagittal MRI image; **f**: postcontrast T1 weighted coronal MRI image)

injure the thalamostriate veins or the fornices during such operations. Also, more caution should be exercised in operating on the lateral ventricle on the dominant side, as the risks are much higher. Residual, recurrent, or asymptomatic tumors can be treated with Gamma Knife.

Tumors of the Third Ventricle

The most common primary third ventricular tumors that can be seen in adults are colloid cysts.

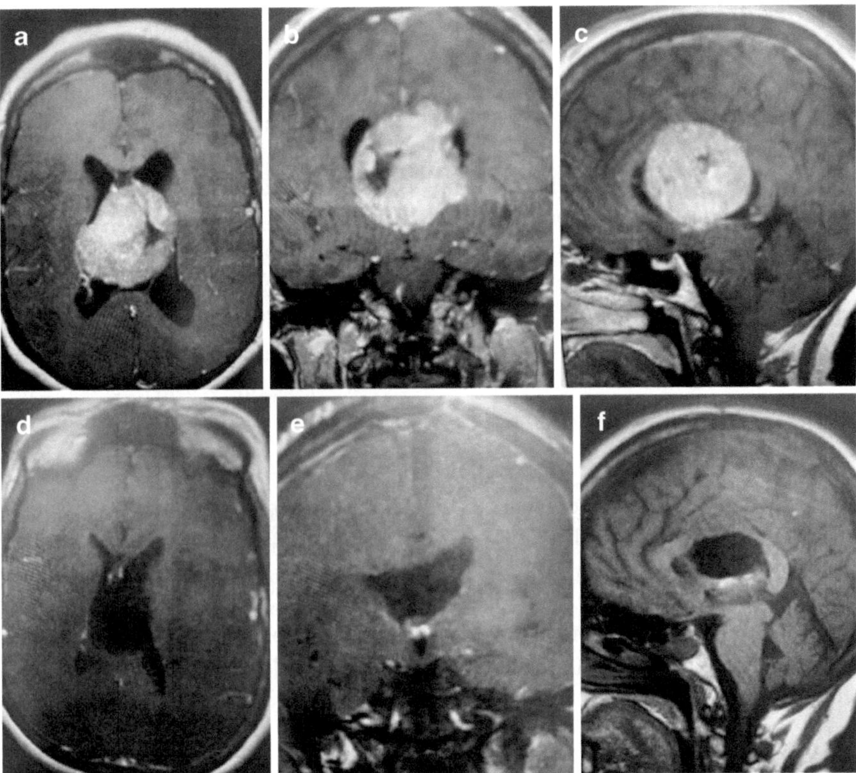

Fig. 7.27 This is a 62-year-old woman who presented with gait instability, leg weakness, visions problems, urinary incontinence, and memory problems. She was found to have a very large meningioma filling both lateral ventricles (**a**: postcontrast T1 axial MRI image; **b**: postcontrast T1 coronal MRI image; **c**: postcontrast T1 sagittal MRI image). Her tumor was removed via a right frontal craniotomy with a transcortical approach using the Vycor tubular retractor and the operating microscope. No shunt was needed. Postoperatively her symptoms improved. Postoperative MRI showed the tumor had been completely removed (**d**: postcontrast T1 axial MRI image; **e**: postcontrast T1 coronal MRI image; **f**: postcontrast T1 sagittal MRI image)

The most common tumors to grow secondarily into the third ventricle in adults are craniopharyngiomas (that can grow secondarily into the anterior third ventricle) and pineal tumors (that can grow secondarily into the posterior third ventricle).

Surgery is appropriate in adults with large, symptomatic craniopharyngiomas, and such tumors often have a large cystic component. The surgical approach usually involves a frontal craniotomy, though sometimes a transsphenoidal approach is reasonable. Radiation or radiosurgery may be appropriate for surgical residual, recurrences, or smaller tumors. During surgery, it is critical not to cause excessive manipulation of the optic nerves or hypothalamus, as injury to these structures can cause serious neurological deficits. It is better to leave adherent tumor and address any residual with radiation.

Tumors of the Fourth Ventricle

Ependymomas can be benign or malignant. These are usually operated on via a midline suboccipital craniectomy approach. It is important not to be overaggressive with the floor of the fourth ventricle which is also the dorsal surface of the brainstem. Adjuvant radiation or chemotherapy may be needed and a spine MRI survey for drop metastases is appropriate.

Subependymomas are benign indolent tumors. They can often be managed with observation or Gamma Knife. If these tumors are causing hydrocephalus, surgical removal via a midline suboccipital approach is appropriate.

Hemangioblastoma

These are benign brain tumors that can develop in the cerebellum. They are usually cystic and contain a mural nodule that is somewhat vascular. These tumors are sometimes associated with Von Hippel Lindau (VHL) syndrome, an autosomal dominant genetic disorder, and one of the phakomatoses/neurocutaneous syndromes. Treatment of symptomatic cerebellar hemangioblastoma is with suboccipital craniectomy and surgical excision of the cyst and nodule (see Fig. 7.28). Residual, recurrent, or asymptomatic tumors can be treated with Gamma Knife [61].

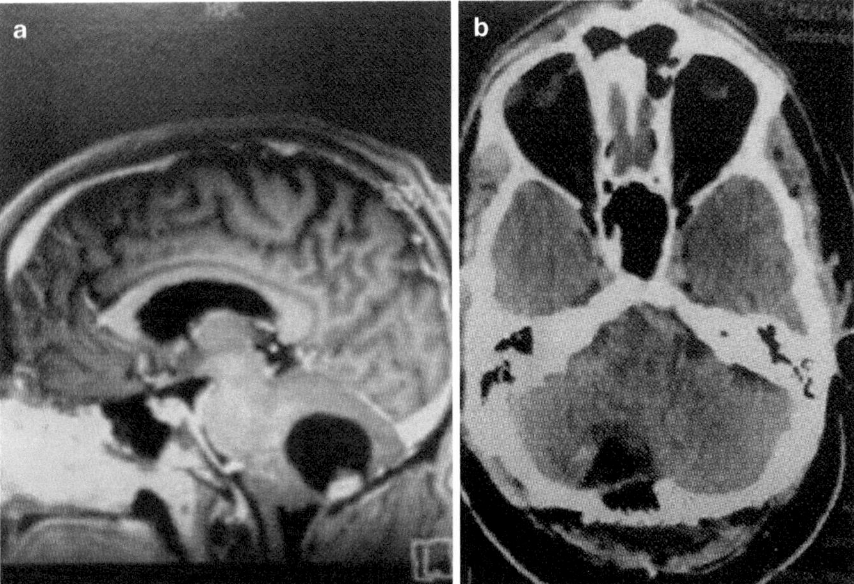

Fig. 7.28 This is a 58-year-old man who presented with several months of progressive right-sided occipital headaches. He was experiencing dizziness at times and felt his coordination was off. He felt his gait was also somewhat abnormal. MRI showed a 4 cm right cerebellar cyst with an associated enhancing mural nodule (**a**: postcontrast T1 sagittal MRI image). He underwent stereotactic guided right suboccipital craniectomy with removal of the cyst and the nodule. Postoperatively, the patient felt better, with complete resolution of his symptoms. Postoperative images showed the cyst and mass were gone (**b**: axial CT image). Pathology showed hemangioblastoma. Work-up for Von Hippel Lindau syndrome was negative, and 3 years later, MRI showed no sign of recurrence

Chapter 8
Brain Cysts

Arachnoid Cysts

These are cysts whose walls are arachnoid and are filled with CSF. They are likely congenital. Sometimes, there can be growth over time. It is extremely rare that an adult with an arachnoid cyst of the brain would require surgical intervention. Often the only symptom reported in patients found to have an arachnoid cyst is "headache," but this is usually unrelated, as headaches are very common in the general population (see Fig. 8.1).

There are rare large symptomatic arachnoid cysts that might benefit from surgical intervention [62]—usually fenestration into normal CSF spaces, such as cisterns or ventricles—but these would be, by far, the exception. Arachnoid cysts of the brain in adults almost never need surgery.

M. H. Brisman, *Put Down the Knife*,
https://doi.org/10.1007/978-3-031-48499-5_8

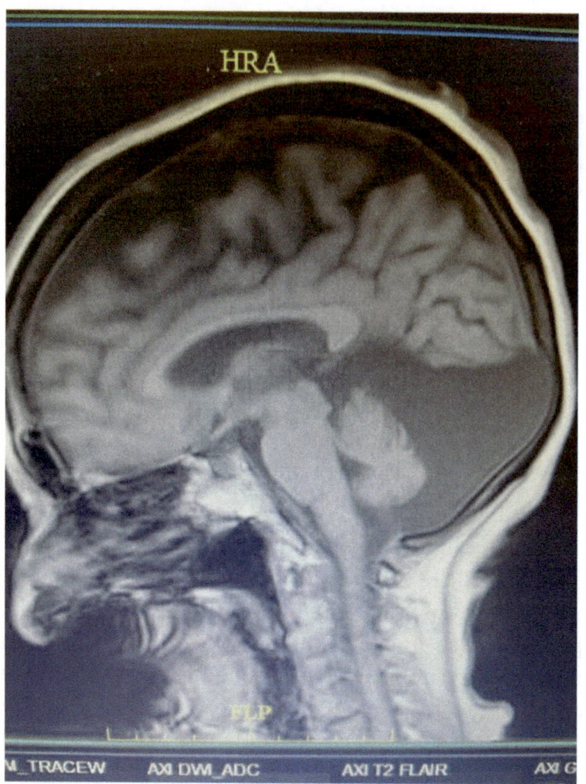

Fig. 8.1 This is a 74-year-old woman with a longstanding history of migraine headaches. She would get about one headache per year. For the past several weeks, she was experiencing a new type of pain in the back of her head, bad headaches primarily in the left occipital region. The pain would sometimes feel like it radiated to the upper neck. MRI of the brain showed a very large arachnoid cyst in the posterior fossa. Her exam was normal. She described her occipital headaches as sudden, sharp, severe twinges of pain that she would get several times per day. Her symptoms were felt to be most consistent with occipital neuralgia, and the arachnoid cyst was felt to be incidental. The patient was started on carbamazepine 50 mg twice a day. Within days, her occipital pain had completely resolved

Pituitary Cysts

Small benign cysts are not uncommon within the pituitary gland. These can almost always just be left alone.

Rathke's Cysts

These are cysts can also develop within the pituitary gland. These cysts are filled with a mucoid-like material. These can also usually be left alone and observed. If these become very large and are causing symptoms, such as vision loss, transsphenoidal endoscopic surgery would be reasonable. But this is rare. If a Rathke's cyst is enlarging and not causing many symptoms, Gamma Knife can be performed.

Pineal Cysts

These are also benign cysts, likely congenital, that can appear in the pineal region. Again, these rarely cause any symptoms and can usually be left alone. Surgery is rarely needed, though would be appropriate in the case of a large, symptomatic pineal cyst. Again, though, this should be rare.

Colloid Cysts

These are cysts that are filled with a mucoid-like material that develop in the third ventricle, in the midline, by the entrance of the foramina of Monroe. Smaller, incidental cysts can be followed or treated with Gamma Knife, depending on the size or growth. Larger colloid cysts that are causing symptoms, often hydrocephalus, should be removed, often urgently. The technically most straightforward surgical approach is the right frontal transcortical approach, guided with neuronavigation, through a small tubular retractor, with the use of the microscope (see Fig. 8.2). It is critical not to pull on the cyst as this can cause bilateral fornix injury and memory problems.

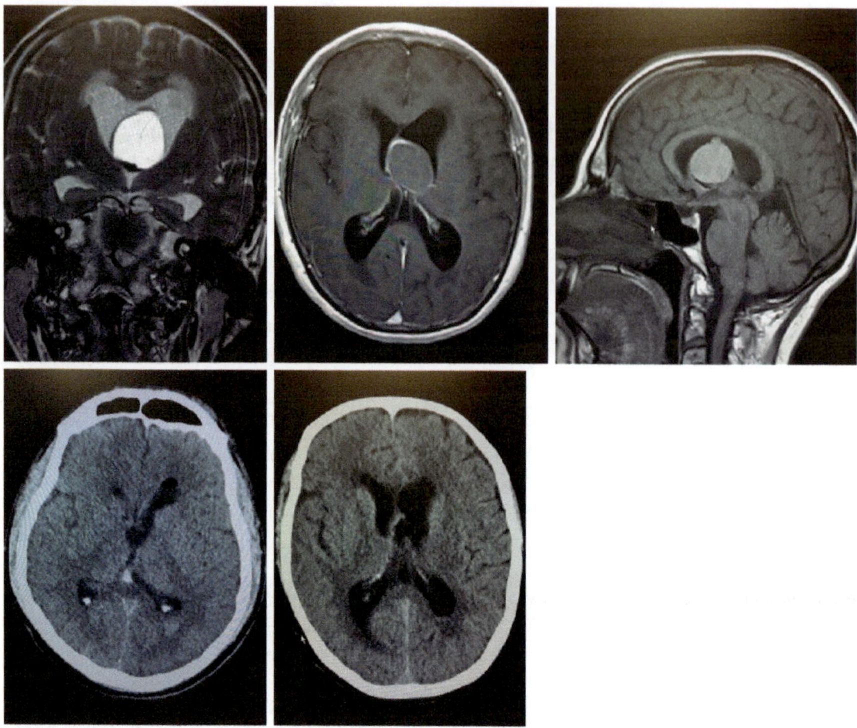

Fig. 8.2 This is a 55-year-old woman who presented with headaches and lethargy found to have a large intraventricular cystic mass, consistent with a colloid cyst of the third ventricle (**a**: coronal T2 weighted MRI image; **b**: postcontrast T1 axial MRI image; **c**: T1 sagittal MRI image). The mass was removed via a left frontal craniotomy, with a transcortical approach, using the Vycor tubular retractor and the operating microscope. The patient made a full recovery. A shunt was not needed. Pathology confirmed a colloid cyst. Postoperative images showed good removal of the mass (**d**, **e**: axial CT image)

Neuroglial Cysts

These cysts can develop in the brain parenchyma. They rarely require treatment. However, if they are large and symptomatic, they can be fenestrated into the cisterns or an adjacent ventricle (with guidance of neuronavigation; see Fig. 8.3).

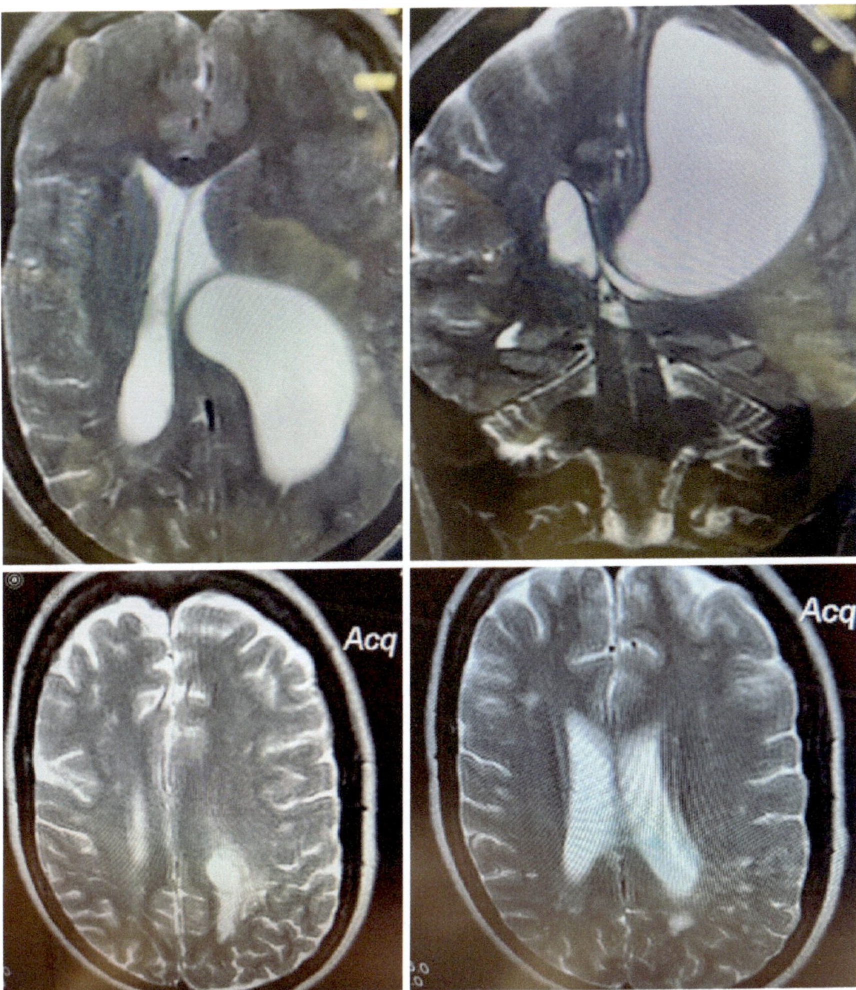

Fig. 8.3 This is a 63-year-old woman with headaches and new balance problems who had an enlarging left parietal-occipital neuroglial cyst that was now causing significant mass effect and midline shift (**a**: T2 weighted axial MRI image; **b**: T2 weighted coronal MRI image). A left parietal craniotomy was performed with stereotactic neuronavigation and the cyst was fenestrated into the left lateral ventricle. Postoperatively, the patient's symptoms resolved. Postoperative MRI imaging showed the cyst was dramatically smaller (**c**: T2 weighted axial MRI image; **d**: T2 weighted axial MRI image, inferior cut)

Chapter 9
Hydrocephalus

Symptomatic hydrocephalus, whether communicating or non-communicating, in an otherwise healthy and viable patient, is a clear indication for neurosurgical intervention. This classic form of hydrocephalus causes high intracranial pressure, and a deteriorating neurological exam, that can ultimately lead to death if not treated. Typical symptoms include bad headaches, nausea, vomiting, confusion, lethargy, and obtundation. There can also be visual impairment or a sixth nerve palsy. Treatments can include ventriculostomy, if the hydrocephalus is expected to be transient, or a shunt. The generally preferred shunting technique is a right frontal ventriculoperitoneal shunt, as the frontal entry site and the peritoneal distal sites are associated with the fewest complications. A 7 cm right angled ventricular catheter will prevent inadvertent deep or shallow placement of the catheter. The neuronavigation system helps to optimize the placement of the ventricular catheter, and a general surgeon can place the peritoneal catheter laparoscopically (usually through a small incision in the umbilicus) [63]. A programmable shunt valve is also usually desirable. Occipital shunts may be reserved for bald men for whom the frontal shunt valve placement would be cosmetically undesirable.

If a patient with a shunt presents with multiple episodes of what seem to be recurrent shunt infections that are otherwise unexplained, which can include redness over the shunt equipment or wound drainage, the rare diagnosis of silicone allergy should be entertained. Replacement of the shunt with a silicone-free shunt will fix this problem.

In the event the hydrocephalus is due to an obstruction within the ventricular system—in the posterior third ventricle, the aqueduct, or the fourth ventricle—an endoscopic third ventriculostomy (ETV) can be performed instead of a shunt.

In rare cases, a patient can develop many of the same symptoms of "classic" hydrocephalus with normal or even low intraventricular pressures (usually after an intracranial hemorrhage or chronic shunting). These patients also require shunting, but with either low pressure valves or programmable valves set to low pressures. Consideration might also be given here to using a lumbar proximal shunt site (in

M. H. Brisman, *Put Down the Knife*,
https://doi.org/10.1007/978-3-031-48499-5_9

cases of communicating hydrocephalus) and/or a pleural distal shunt site. These patients are very challenging to manage and have a significantly poorer prognosis than patients with typical high-pressure hydrocephalus.

Normal Pressure Hydrocephalus (NPH)

This entity is entirely different from "classic" hydrocephalus. In this entity, patients, usually elderly patients in their 60s and 70s, are found to have enlarged ventricles (ventriculomegaly) and associated symptoms that include gait difficulty and may also include memory impairment and/or urinary incontinence. If a lumbar puncture is performed, the pressure is found to be normal.

The problem here is that many elderly patients have enlarged ventricles (due mostly to atrophy) and some gait difficulties or memory loss or urinary incontinence. Nursing homes are likely full of such patients. Yet very few people who have these features will actually benefit from a ventriculoperitoneal shunt. Perhaps a distinction should be made between the term "normal pressure hydrocephalus," which defines a condition of enlarged ventricles with normal pressure that are causing neurological symptoms and, the much more common "normal pressure ventriculomegaly," which could define a condition of enlarged ventricles with normal pressure that are not suspected of causing neurological symptoms.

Shunts in these NPH cases are reportedly most beneficial when the gait and memory problems are fairly mild to begin with. Of note, many of these potential surgical candidates are not that bothered by their mild walking issues or their mild memory issues and have little interest in any brain operation. It is also not completely clear why a shunt would help in these cases. The shunt presumably does not drain much fluid as the pressure is normal to begin with, and follow-up imaging often shows no change in ventricular size. Perhaps some patients with NPH who benefit from medium pressure shunts have high/normal intracranial pressures.

Even for those patients who are reportedly better with a shunt, the improvements are often very subtle and can be documented only with detailed testing. Furthermore, many of these patients, at long-term follow-up after shunting, will show minimal improvement, no improvement, or worsening of their clinical conditions. One analysis that reviewed 44 publications showed only 29% of shunted patients experienced prolonged or significant improvement [64]. This same study showed a 38% complication rate, a 22% rate of re-operation, and a 6% rate of major complication or death. A more recent study showed that of patients shunted for NPH, only 43% had a clinically significant improvement in health-related quality of life at 1 year follow-up [65]. Another study showed little difference at long-term follow-up between such patients who were shunted compared with those who were not shunted [66].

There is also some evidence that patients suspected of having NPH might benefit from oral acetazolamide (a medicine that decreases CSF production), just like patients with idiopathic intracranial hypertension. One study showed many patients with presumed NPH improved with oral acetazolamide, and that there was often persistent benefit at 1 year follow-up [67]. Another small study also showed many patients with presumed NPH improved with acetazolamide, and that patients who improved showed a significant decrease in the volume of periventricular white matter hyperintensity volume [68]. Further study of acetazolamide in this context would make sense.

All that said, criteria for even considering a shunt surgery for possible NPH should be stringent and should include (1) the patient has clearly enlarged ventricles in the presence of limited generalized brain atrophy; (2) the patient has few confounding medical co-morbidities; (3) the patient has insidious onset of mild to moderate gait difficulties and possibly memory problems or urinary incontinence that have no other obvious explanations as to their cause; and (4) the patient shows dramatic improvement of their symptoms after a high volume lumbar puncture (see Fig. 9.1). At the very least, more study is needed here to better select the patients who will significantly benefit from shunt operations.

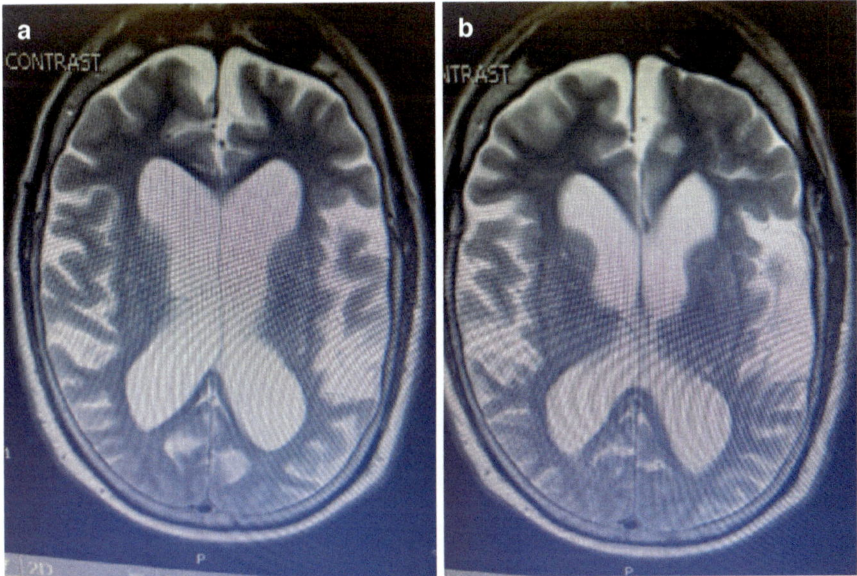

Fig. 9.1 This is a 70-year-old man with the main complaint of some mild intermittent memory issues for about a year. He also had periodic imbalance for several years. He had spinal stenosis and episodes of pain radiating down his legs that had improved with epidural steroid injections. He also had very rare mild episodes of urinary incontinence. Brain MRI (**a**, **b**) showed enlarged ventricles and moderate diffuse brain atrophy that was unchanged compared with an MRI from 6 years earlier. Medical history was also noteworthy for hypertension being treated with multiple medicines and trigeminal neuralgia controlled on a low dose of carbamazepine (200 mg BID). After consultation, the patient's carbamazepine was switched to gabapentin. The patient quickly noted a significant improvement in his alertness and his memory. He did not wish to pursue a diagnostic spinal tap

Idiopathic Intracranial Hypertension

Also known as "pseudotumor cerebri," this condition involves high pressures in the brain without any discernable mass. It frequently affects young, overweight women and can cause headaches, papilledema, and visual loss. A common cause is thought to be a narrowed transverse sinus, and sinus stenting is another consideration in refractory cases. Usually, this condition can be managed with acetazolamide and weight loss. For patients with deteriorating vision or intractable headaches despite medicines, a shunt can be offered. A right frontal VP shunt can be placed with neuronavigational guidance, unless the ventricles are very small, in which case a lumbo-peritoneal shunt can be offered. Surgery is rarely needed in this condition.

Chapter 10
Pain Disorders

Trigeminal Neuralgia

This disease involves intermittent, sudden, brief, severe, sharp (electric shock or stabbing) pains in the face (in the trigeminal distribution), which are usually triggered by light touch and usually respond to carbamazepine or oxcarbazepine. The pains are often described as "shooting" or "radiating" in nature. There can also be a minor component of constant achy pains in the trigeminal distribution. Spontaneous remissions are common. The definition of trigeminal neuralgia as any idiopathic spontaneous facial pain, subcategorized as TN1 if such pain is predominantly episodic and TN2 if it is predominantly constant, is not advisable. Such a broad definition will, necessarily, include many patients who clearly do not have true trigeminal neuralgia and will not likely benefit from the standard trigeminal neuralgia procedures (microvascular decompression/MVD or trigeminal denervation). Of note, if a patient experiences clear dramatic pain relief after one of the standard trigeminal neuralgia procedures, that suggests that trigeminal neuralgia was probably the correct diagnosis.

Trigeminal neuralgia should specifically be distinguished from post-herpetic neuralgia (which follows a shingles rash outbreak, usually in a V1 distribution, and often involves numbness and a predominantly constant achy pain), nerve injury pain (which can follow from some nerve injury, such as might be caused by dental work, and often involves numbness and a predominantly constant achy pain), and chronic paroxysmal hemicrania (in which the pain usually centers in and around the eye, involves autonomic features, and is very responsive to Indomethacin). Trigeminal neuralgia should also be distinguished from other types of idiopathic neuropathic facial pains (sometimes called "atypical facial pain") that are usually more constant and achier or burning in nature and are usually best treated with medicine and conservative management (see Case 10.1).

M. H. Brisman, *Put Down the Knife*,
https://doi.org/10.1007/978-3-031-48499-5_10

Case 10.1

This is a 41-year-old man with 15 years of intermittent pains in the right side of his face. He was otherwise healthy. The pains would come on every day. They occurred in the right jaw and could radiate back toward the ear. At times, the pain would radiate toward the neck and toward the left side. Flexeril and Xanax did not help. When he got the pain, he felt that taking ibuprofen prevented the pains from getting worse. The pains were achy, dull pains, about 4/10 in severity, on a scale of 1–10. The pains would develop gradually over hours and usually occurred in the afternoons. Exam was normal and brain MRI was unremarkable. This was felt to be a neuropathic facial pain. He was started on gabapentin 200 mg TID. His pain was completely resolved by the medicine.

Trigeminal neuralgia is usually caused by a blood vessel, usually an artery, contacting or compressing the trigeminal nerve root. It can also be caused by multiple sclerosis, or a brain mass contacting the trigeminal nerve root. Sometimes, no cause can be found. The first line treatment is with the antiseizure medicines carbamazepine or oxcarbazepine. Gabapentin is usually used as the second line medicine. Other antiseizure medicines can also be used. Dilantin is useful for acute uncontrolled pain in the emergency room because it can be loaded quickly. Work-up for trigeminal neuralgia is with a brain MRI. A fine cut T2 weighted sequence (FIESTA or CISS) may demonstrate the offending blood vessel. That said, vascular contact against the trigeminal nerve (or the facial or glossopharyngeal nerves for that matter) is a common occurrence and in no way confirms the diagnosis of a cranial nerve hyperactivity syndrome such as trigeminal neuralgia. Furthermore, a significant neuro-vascular contact can be present that is not fully appreciated on FIESTA imaging, and lack of "definitive" vascular compression should not discourage the performance of an MVD in an otherwise appropriate operative candidate.

For those patients for whom medicines do not adequately control the pain, or for whom the side effects of the medicines are not tolerable, a procedure is appropriate (microvascular decompression, percutaneous rhizotomy, or radiosurgery). Of note, one of the trigeminal neuralgia procedures is not likely to help a patient who has a facial pain syndrome other than trigeminal neuralgia. The microvascular decompression (MVD) is a good choice for younger patients (under about 65–70), who are healthy and do not have multiple sclerosis [69]. MVD is more likely to be effective if the offending vessel is an artery (usually the superior cerebellar artery) and is more likely to be successful if the offending artery was distorting the nerve. Neuronavigation is helpful in identifying the transverse-sigmoid junction. Intradurally, the petrosal vein can be sacrificed, if needed. The use of brain retractors should be avoided as this increases the chance of an eighth nerve injury. Furthermore, neuromonitoring changes of either the eighth or seventh nerve during the micro-dissection suggest an imminent retraction injury to the eighth nerve and should prompt the surgeon to pause and then redirect the surgical activity. An endoscope can sometimes enhance the view, particularly distally toward the entrance of Meckel's cave. Veins contacting the trigeminal nerve can be cauterized and divided, but caution must be taken not to injure the nerve itself through a heating effect. Ideally at the end of the MVD procedure, there will be no blood vessels or implants (like Teflon felt) contacting the trigeminal nerve (see Figs. 10.1 and 10.2). Repeat MVDs should usually be avoided. The risk for repeat MVDs is much higher due to scarring, and postoperative pain relief that is obtained is frequently due to denervation, so these operations are generally no more than open rhizotomies.

Recent considerations for avoiding the use of Teflon felt during MVD are not unreasonable, as the felt itself often causes an aseptic meningitis (though this can usually be minimized by putting patients on a tapering 3-week course of dexamethasone after the surgery). If at the time of MVD no clear offending vessel is found, the nerve can be injured slightly by gently massaging the nerve or making two tiny grooves in the surface of the nerve with a micro-dissector (a modified combing technique). An "open rhizotomy" can be performed in the same way, in the rare case that the less invasive denervating techniques are not successful.

For older patients, patients with serious medical problems, patients with multiple sclerosis, patients who have already had an MVD, and patients who just prefer a less invasive alternative, a denervating procedure (such as percutaneous rhizotomy or Gamma Knife) is reasonable.

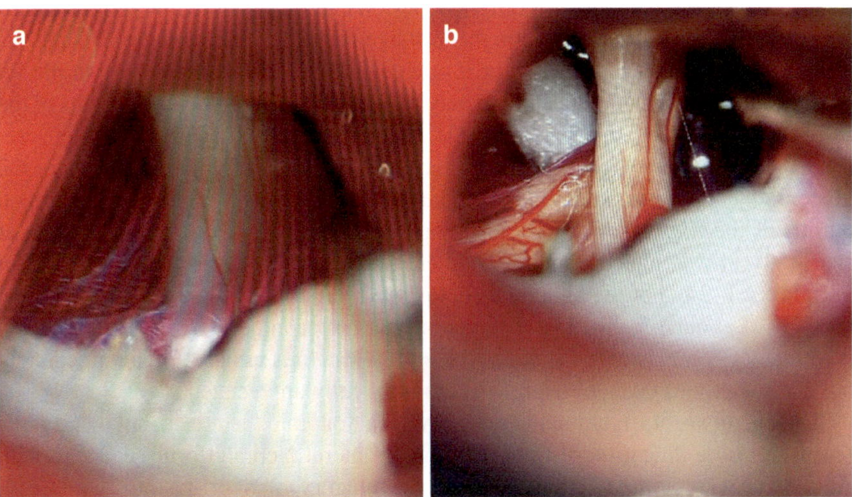

Fig. 10.1 This is a 62-year-old man with right-sided trigeminal neuralgia that was refractory to medical and conservative measures. Intra-operative view under the surgical microscope showing the loop of the superior cerebellar artery coursing along the pons and compressing and flattening the trigeminal nerve at the root entry zone (**a**). After the artery has been moved away toward the tentorium with Teflon felt, the trigeminal nerve is noted to be completely decompressed (**b**). The patient had immediate and lasting relief from his trigeminal neuralgia pain

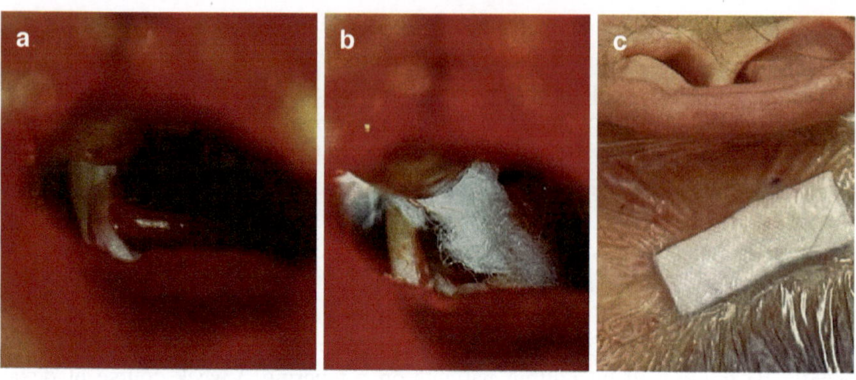

Fig. 10.2 This is a 59-year-old woman with left-sided trigeminal neuralgia who had failed medical and conservative measures. This was the view under microscope of her MVD. At surgery, a loop of the superior cerebellar artery was noted to be significantly compressing the trigeminal nerve root (**a**). The artery was separated from the nerve with micro-dissectors and pushed away with a piece of Teflon felt (**b**). The entire operation was done through an incision about 1.5 inches long (**c**). Postoperatively, the patient's pain was gone and has remained so

For percutaneous rhizotomy, the radiofrequency, glycerol, or balloon techniques can all be used [70, 71], and it is good practice for the surgeon to be prepared and set up to do any of these, depending on the circumstances during surgery (see Fig. 10.3). When the rhizotomy is performed, placement of a small metal marker over the middle of either ear can help confirm that the fluoroscopy is shooting a true lateral skull image. For radiofrequency lesioning, one lesion can be performed at 65–75° centigrade for 50–90 s. The need for higher voltage during testing stimulation suggests the need for higher temperatures for lesion generation. If the pain is only in the V3 distribution, a down curved electrode may be used. Intraoperative assessments of the extent of denervation are often unreliable. Radiofrequency is usually not used to create V1 lesions as this technique has a higher likelihood of causing keratitis. For the glycerol injection, it is preferable to see good CSF flow from the cannula and a good outline of the trigeminal cistern during an omnipaque injection. About 0.25 cc of sterile glycerol is injected with the patient sitting upright, and the patient is kept upright for 1–2 h. For the balloon technique, the balloon is inflated for 60–90 s to a pressure of about 1.5 atm. The glycerol or balloon techniques are preferred if there is a large V1 component to the pain. Rhizotomy benefit is usually noted immediately but can sometimes take up to a few weeks to be fully appreciated.

The diagnosis of trigeminal neuralgia with autonomic features is not clearly different from the diagnosis of Short-lasting Unilateral Neuralgiform headache with Autonomic symptoms (SUNA) and the subcategory of Short-lasting, Unilateral, Neuralgiform headache attacks with Conjunctival injection and Tearing (SUNCT). These may just be variants of the same disease [72, 73]. That said, these must be distinguished from chronic paroxysmal hemicrania (another "trigeminal autonomic cephalgia"), which involves sharp attacks of pain in and around the eye, with autonomic features, and complete response to Indomethacin (with poor response to carbamazepine and other anticonvulsants; see Case 10.2).

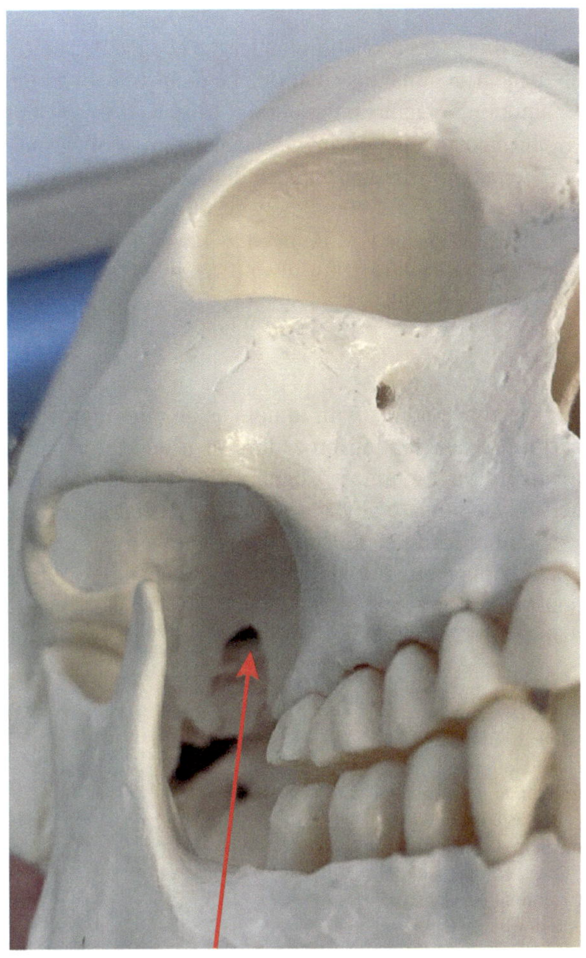

Fig. 10.3 A right-sided skull model with demonstration of access to the foramen ovale for purposes of a percutaneous trigeminal rhizotomy

Case 10.2

This is a 51-year-old woman who presented with 3 years of worsening episodes of severe right facial pain. The pain was in and around the eye. The pain was initially more of a dull pain but was now characterized as primarily sharp intermittent pains. She also had some burning and throbbing pains that were not as bad or bothersome for her. Her pain was described as a stabbing pain that could be triggered by light touch or the wind. The pain could be severe and had brought the patient several times to the emergency room. She referred to her pains as a "raging" of her face. MRI of the brain was unremarkable. She felt she might have gotten slight relief from carbamazepine, but not significant relief of pain. Gabapentin had also not helped with the pain. She noted at times tearing of the right eye and a right nasal drip. She also noted at times that there was a swelling under the eye itself. The sudden, sharp, severe pains in the trigeminal distribution, the focus of pain around the eye, the presence of autonomic features, the normal MRI, and the lack of response to carbamazepine and gabapentin suggested a diagnosis of chronic paroxysmal hemicrania. The patient was started on Indomethacin 25 mg orally twice a day. Her pain immediately and completely resolved, but the medicine bothered her stomach. The dosage was reduced to 15 mg BID, and she had excellent pain control with no side effects. Over time, she was able to taper off the indomethacin and restart it when the pain episodes would flare up.

For most patients with tumors as an etiology of the pain, it is usually easier to perform a denervating procedure, if needed, for pain control, and a radiosurgery treatment for the tumor. A denervating procedure is also preferred if the trigeminal nerve is compressed by a large ectatic basilar artery (see Fig. 10.4).

Gamma Knife can also be an effective treatment for trigeminal neuralgia [74]. For Gamma Knife initial treatments, 80 Gy to the 100% isodose line can be used for non-MS patients, and 85 Gy to the 100% isodose line for MS patients, with no more than the 20% isodose line touching the brainstem. For repeat treatments,

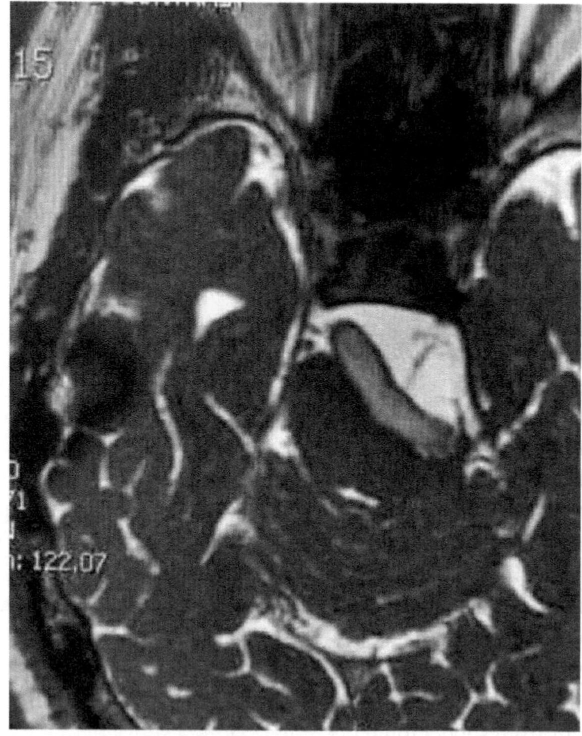

Fig. 10.4 This is a 40-year-old man with classic left-sided trigeminal neuralgia. His pain was controlled on medicines. Brain imaging showed compression of the trigeminal nerve and left anterior brainstem by a very large ectatic basilar artery (T2 axial MRI image). If medical management were to fail, an MVD would not be a good choice here

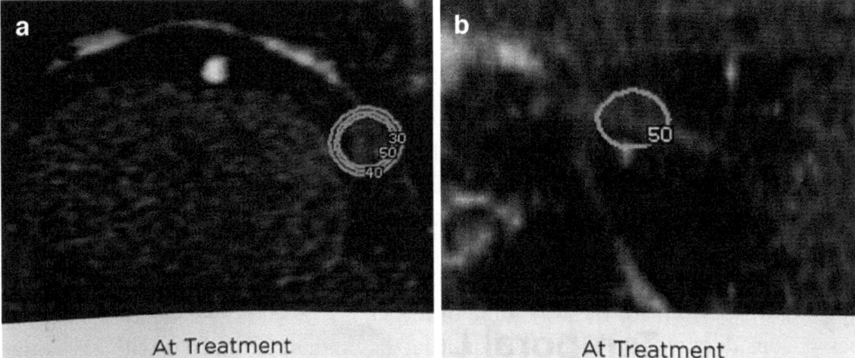

Fig. 10.5 This is a 60-year-old man with medically refractory trigeminal neuralgia in a left V2 distribution. He had an unsuccessful percutaneous rhizotomy elsewhere. He had a history of coronary artery disease and a triple bypass. Gamma Knife was performed (**a**: postcontrast T1 axial image during Gamma Knife treatment; **b**: postcontrast T1 sagittal reconstructed image during Gamma Knife treatment). Fourteen years later, he remains pain free, with no numbness, and requiring no medicines. Note, that my current treatments involve targeting the nerve a bit farther from the brainstem

appropriate doses range anywhere from 40 to 75 Gy to the 100% isodose line depending on the circumstances including time from the last Gamma Knife treatment and the degree of current facial numbness (see Fig. 10.5).

While either denervating procedure (rhizotomy or Gamma Knife) can be repeated, caution should be used in the timing of repeat Gamma Knife procedures as the full effect of these procedures can take quite a while to manifest itself. As such, it is ideal to wait at least 2 years between Gamma Knife trigeminal nerve treatments, including 2 years between treatment of the trigeminal nerve itself and an adjacent tumor (and vice versa).

It is critical not to underestimate the potential bothersomeness of excessive trigeminal denervation. Facial numbness, dysesthesias, and achy pains can be very bothersome to patients (as can medicines, for that matter). Furthermore, numbness of the eye can lead to keratitis and even blindness and should be treated with frequent use of eye drops and regular visits with an ophthalmologist. Ultimately, the real issue is whether the denervation effects are perceived as a problem for the individual patient. While these effects often do lessen over time, it can often take a year or more for such an improvement to occur. As such, it is better to err on the side of creating too little denervation than too much, as further denervation can always be performed at a later time.

Glossopharyngeal Neuralgia

This rare condition has similar features to trigeminal neuralgia but involves the ninth cranial nerve. These patients may experience sudden, brief, severe, sharp pains in their deep ear or throat, triggered by light touch, and relieved with carbamazepine. Like trigeminal neuralgia, this disease is thought to usually be caused by compression of a blood vessel against the ninth cranial nerve. For younger patients who have failed medical management, an MVD is preferred [75], and for older patients, or patients with significant medical co-morbidities, a Gamma Knife procedure can be performed. If, at the time of MVD, no vessel is seen against the ninth nerve, consideration can be given to injuring the ninth nerve slightly with a massaging or combing technique. While cutting the ninth nerve (and possibly the upper one or two branches of the tenth nerve) is considered acceptable in these situations, such action should be taken only with great hesitancy as this can cause significant side effects that are bothersome to the patient, including dysesthesias and deafferentation pain (see Fig. 10.6).

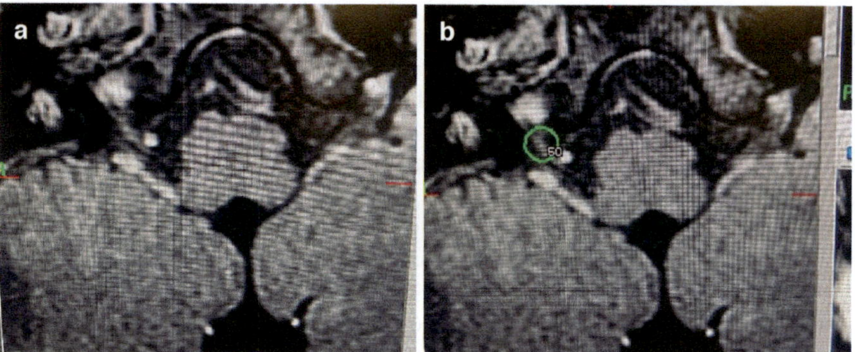

Fig. 10.6 This is a 22-year-old man with autism who is nonverbal. For the past year, he had experienced what seemed to be sudden severe episodes of pain in the right ear that lasted a few minutes and then would go away. Ear exam was normal. The pain was initially better on gabapentin, but he now had to increase his dose 3600 mg/day and was still having episodes of pain. He also still had pain episodes when carbamazepine was added. MRI showed a medium-sized artery contacting the right ninth cranial nerve. Because it was not possible for the patient to confirm the exact nature of his symptoms, it was decided to try a Gamma Knife treatment for presumed right glossopharyngeal neuralgia. Several weeks after Gamma Knife treatment, the patient had no more episodes of pain. (**a**) MRI axial postcontrast image at time of Gamma Knife treatment, showing a medium-sized artery contacting the right ninth cranial nerve; (**b**) MRI axial postcontrast image at the time of Gamma Knife treatment with targeting of the ninth nerve

Occipital Neuralgia

This is a condition in which people get sudden, brief, sharp, intermittent, severe pains on one side of the occipital region in the distribution of the occipital nerve. There can also be some constant and some achy component to these pains. The pains may seem to radiate and can be triggered by light touch in the occipital region. Occipital neuralgia can be caused by disease of the occipital nerve, including compressive masses or trauma. Often the cause is not known. Carbamazepine and gabapentin can help relieve these pains. Occipital nerve blocks can also be performed. For refractory cases, occipital nerve decompression in the posterior scalp can be considered. If other treatments are not successful, a trial of a peripheral occipital stimulator can be considered (with permanent internalization if the trial is successful).

Pain Procedures for Other Cranio-facial Pains

The procedures that currently seem to have the most potential are implantation of percutaneous peripheral nerve stimulators in the distribution of either the trigeminal nerve [76] or the occipital nerve [77]. These patients first undergo a trial implant and then permanent implant if the trial is successful. V3 distribution stimulators carry the extra challenge of potential lead migration due to movement of the mandible. These procedures are generally very low risk.

Chapter 11
Movement Disorders

Most people with movement disorders will not benefit from brain surgery. Newer medicines have minimized the need for surgery for such disorders. However, there are a few categories of adult patients with movement disorders who may benefit from brain surgery.

Hemifacial Spasm

Patients with this disorder may have varying degrees of facial spasms and disability. Often the symptoms are mild. In many cases, patients can be managed with various medicines (such as carbamazepine or gabapentin) or with Botox injections (see Fig. 11.1). For those patients with extremely bothersome symptoms who are not satisfied with other treatments, microvascular decompression (MVD) can be curative [78, 79]. The usual cause of the compression is an artery against the facial nerve just as it exits the brainstem (see Fig. 11.2). The major risk of MVD, particularly with hemifacial spasm, is injury to the eighth nerve, with resultant ipsilateral hearing loss or vestibular dysfunction. Also, of late, there has been some thought to avoiding the use of the traditional Teflon felt to avoid the frequent chemical meningitis that the felt often induces. Sometimes, the benefits of the MVD in these cases can take several months to appreciate.

M. H. Brisman, *Put Down the Knife*,
https://doi.org/10.1007/978-3-031-48499-5_11

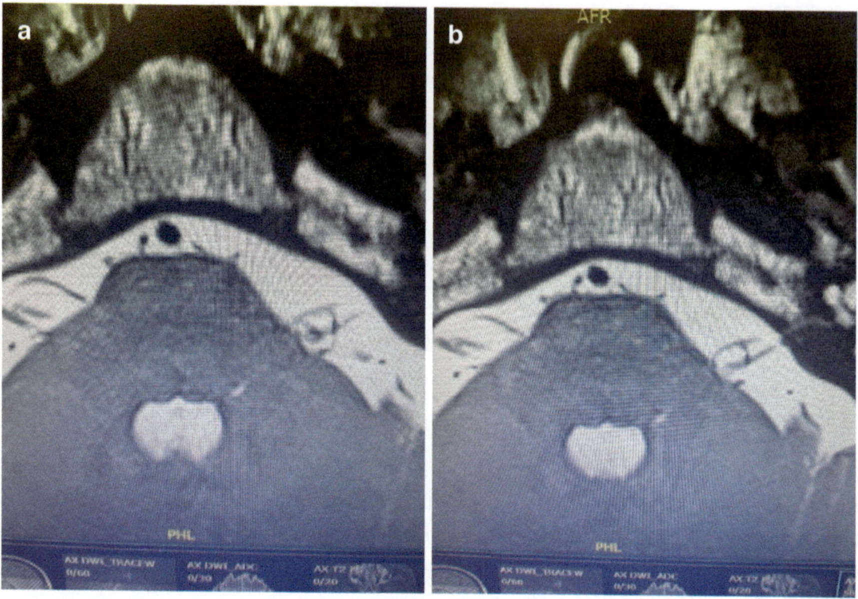

Fig. 11.1 This is a 44-year-old man who had progressive development of severe left-sided hemifacial spasm that involved the entire left side of his face. MRI was ordered which was consistent with an arterial loop compressing and distorting the left facial nerve (**a**, **b**: Fiesta sequence MRI showing left facial nerve compression by an arterial loop). The patient was started on carbamazepine 100 mg TID. His facial twitching dramatically improved. He was very happy and opted to continue on the medicines with no other treatments

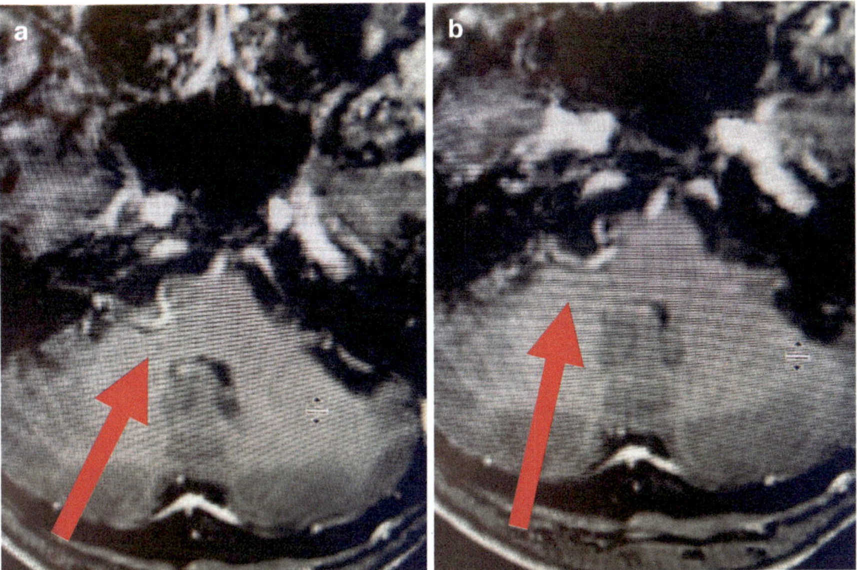

Fig. 11.2 This is a 62-year-old woman with right-sided hemifacial spasm that was severe, bothersome, and refractory to conservative measures. Her MRI shows an artery compressing the facial nerve by the root entry zone (**a**, **b**: postcontrast T1 axial MRI images). The patient underwent an MVD at which time the offending artery was moved away from the facial nerve root with Teflon felt. After several months, her hemifacial spasm completely went away

Tremor

Again, medicines and conservative therapies are almost always the treatment of choice for this condition. However, for severe refractory cases of essential tremor or tremor dominant Parkinson's disease, procedures can be considered and can help, including Gamma Knife thalamotomy [80], MR guided focused ultrasound (MRgFUS) [81, 82], and Deep Brain Stimulation (DBS) [83], though these procedures all carry some rate of serious complication.

Other Movement Disorders

There are other movement disorders, including Parkinson's and dystonias, that are almost always managed with medicines and conservative therapies. Again, though, if symptoms are severe and refractory to other treatments, deep brain stimulation with various targets, including the subthalamic nucleus (STN) [84] and the internal globus pallidus (GPi) [85], can be considered.

Chapter 12
Brain Abscess

These can be caused by various microbes including bacteria, fungi, or parasites. They can result from direct or hematogenous spread. They may be single or multiple. They may be of varying sizes. Certain infections, such as parasitic toxoplasmosis, are more likely in patients who are immunocompromised. Usually, the treatment for brain abscesses is with antimicrobial medicines. Surgery for a brain abscess would be appropriate (1) if the organism was not known or (2) there was one large symptomatic and accessible abscess. In the event drainage is sought, entry is normally from a cortical approach. Neuronavigation is often helpful, as is a tubular retractor if the abscess is deep (see Fig. 12.1).

M. H. Brisman, *Put Down the Knife*,
https://doi.org/10.1007/978-3-031-48499-5_12

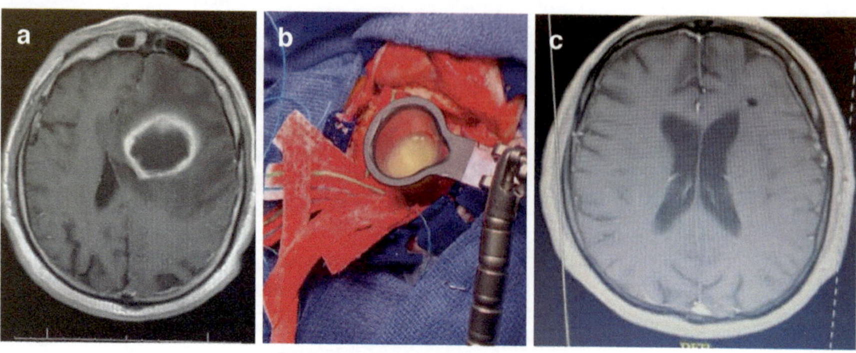

Fig. 12.1 This is a 50-year-old man who last year had undergone a gastrectomy for gastric cancer. He presented now with new onset of lethargy, aphasia (expressive and receptive), and intermittent bradycardia. Brain imaging showed a 3 cm ring enhancing fluid filled mass in the deep left frontal region with significant surrounding edema (**a**: postcontrast T1 axial MRI image). A left frontal craniotomy was performed, using a transcortical approach with stereotactic neuronavigation, through a tubular retractor. Purulent material was encountered under pressure consistent with a brain abscess (**b**). The purulent material was fully washed out with gentle irrigation. The patient was treated with several weeks of broad-spectrum IV antibiotics. Gram stains were suspicious for the presence of bacteria (encapsulated cocci). The patient made a full recovery. Follow-up MRI showed complete resolution of the abscess (**c**: postcontrast T1 axial MRI image)

Chapter 13
Chiari Malformation

These may or may not be accompanied by syringomyelia. These can also rarely be associated with Ehlers Danlos syndrome (EDS). Often Chiari 1 malformations are asymptomatic and can then be managed with observation.

For Chiari 1 malformations that are causing significant symptoms, posterior decompressive surgery is appropriate. The MIST (minimally invasive subpial tonsillectomy) procedure [86] is an excellent option when surgery is needed. It involves a smaller incision, a smaller opening of bone (occiput just 2 cm from the foramen, with just part of the C1 lamina), a linear dural incision, and resection of the cerebellar tonsils. Alternatively, "shrinkage" of the tonsils with a low setting on the cautery system may also be adequate (see Fig. 13.1). Care must be taken not to injure the PICA artery loops or the spinal accessory nerves. Excessively large bone work far from the foramen magnum is not clearly helpful. And while suturing in a large dural patch graft does provide extra intradural room, the patch graft adds time and complexity to the procedure that is not clearly necessary to decompress the foramen magnum and makes pseudomeningoceles and CSF leaks much more likely. Of note, if a Chiari malformation is felt to be secondary to some other condition, such as idiopathic intracranial hypertension, it is usually best to address that primary condition first.

M. H. Brisman, *Put Down the Knife*,
https://doi.org/10.1007/978-3-031-48499-5_13

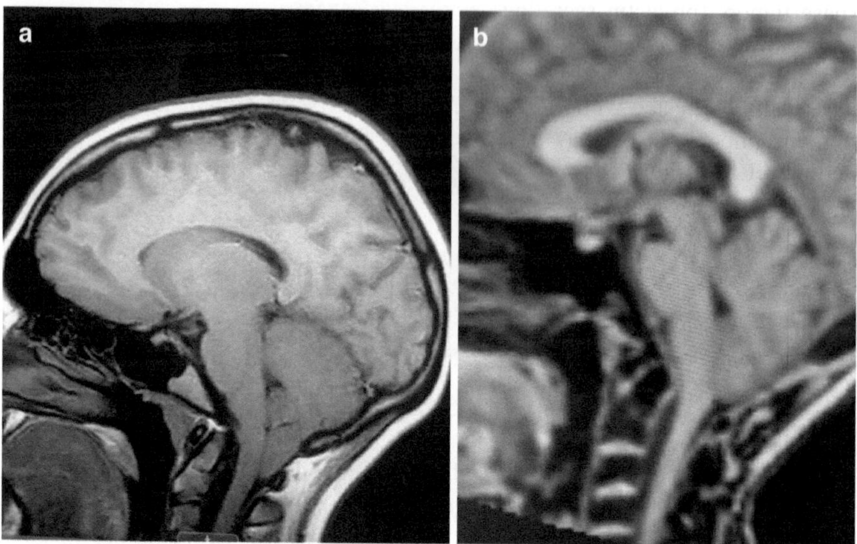

Fig. 13.1 This is a 23-year-old woman with persistent bothersome occipital headaches worse with coughing and straining. MRI showed a Chiari 1 malformation (**a**: sagittal T1 MRI image). The patient underwent suboccipital craniectomy and cerebellar tonsillectomy (MIST procedure). Her pre-operative symptoms resolved. Postoperative MRI showed resection/decompression of cerebellar tonsils (**b**: sagittal T1 MRI image)

Chapter 14
Skull Base Disorders

This subcategory of adult brain surgery generally has the following features: (1) a tumor, benign or malignant, that involves part of the skull base; (2) a complex opening that carries much higher risk than the standard craniotomy openings; (3) dissection of tumor off cranial nerves and critical blood vessels (sometimes even involving sacrifice of such blood vessels or blood vessel bypass procedures); (4) higher risk of a serious complication.

One should specifically exclude from this category minimally invasive "endoscopic endonasal approach" (EEA) procedures for removal of masses such as pituitary adenomas and clival chordomas, and standard cranial approaches to remove olfactory groove, planum sphenoidale, and sphenoid wing meningiomas. One should also exclude any non-invasive management of such problems, such as with Gamma Knife.

The risks of these "skull base operations" are often very high, and the benefits of such procedures are generally significantly less than other alternatives. The major alternative for most of these tumor cases is some form of radiation, whether Gamma Knife, hypofractionated radiosurgery (usually performed in 5 doses), or even just standard focused radiation treatment over the course of several weeks (see Figs. 14.1, 14.2, 14.3, and 14.4). There is rarely any benefit in trying to aggressively dissect a tumor off cranial nerves or critical blood vessels. Whether the tumor is benign or malignant, the tumor control will be just as good with radiosurgery, and the expected neurological deficits with be much less. It is also worth noting that most brain surgeons who specialize in "skull base surgery" (or surgery for other brain tumors, for that matter) are often not that experienced in performing stereotactic radiosurgery and thus may not fully appreciate the benefits of this much less invasive modality. Even larger skull base tumors can often be treated either with hypofractionated or staged radiosurgery techniques, or standard fractionated radiation. As an important general rule, a benign brain tumor can usually be stabilized at its current size and symptomatology with radiation alone.

M. H. Brisman, *Put Down the Knife*,
https://doi.org/10.1007/978-3-031-48499-5_14

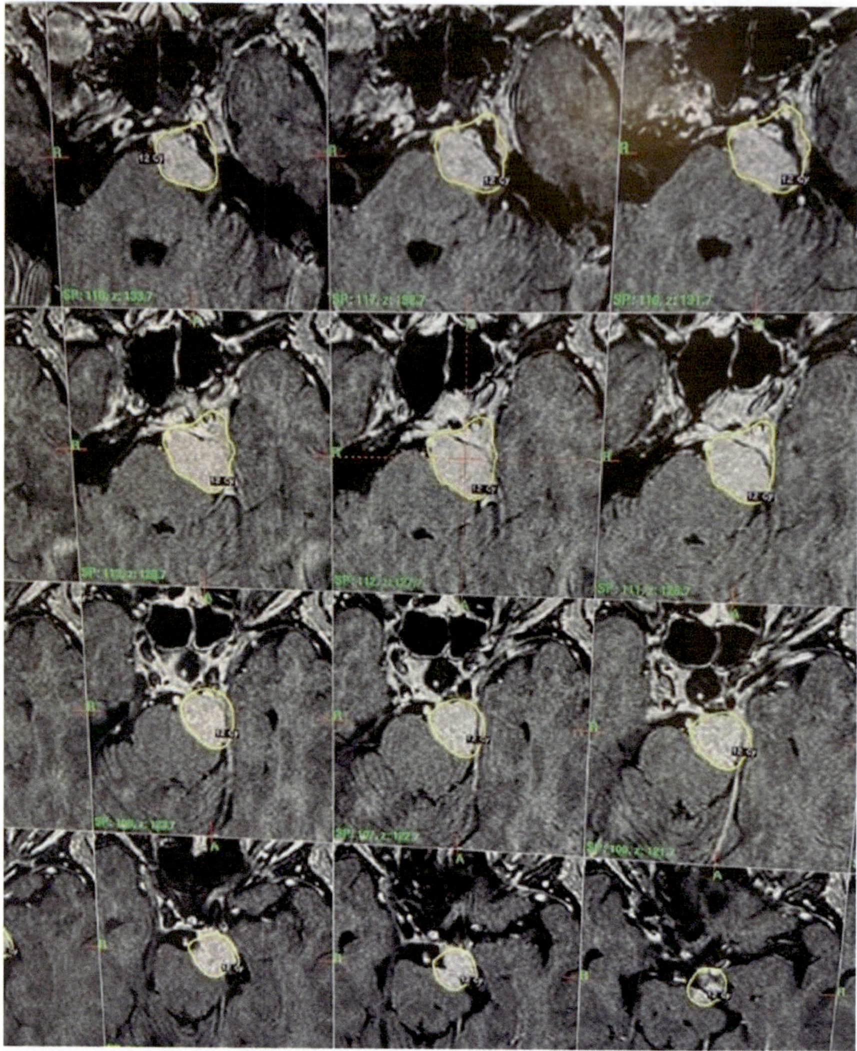

Fig. 14.1 This is a 68-year-old woman found incidentally to have a 2 cm meningioma in the left retroclival/cavernous sinus region, indenting the left anterior brainstem. She was treated with Gamma Knife (postcontrast T1 weighted axial MRI images from the time of Gamma Knife treatment)

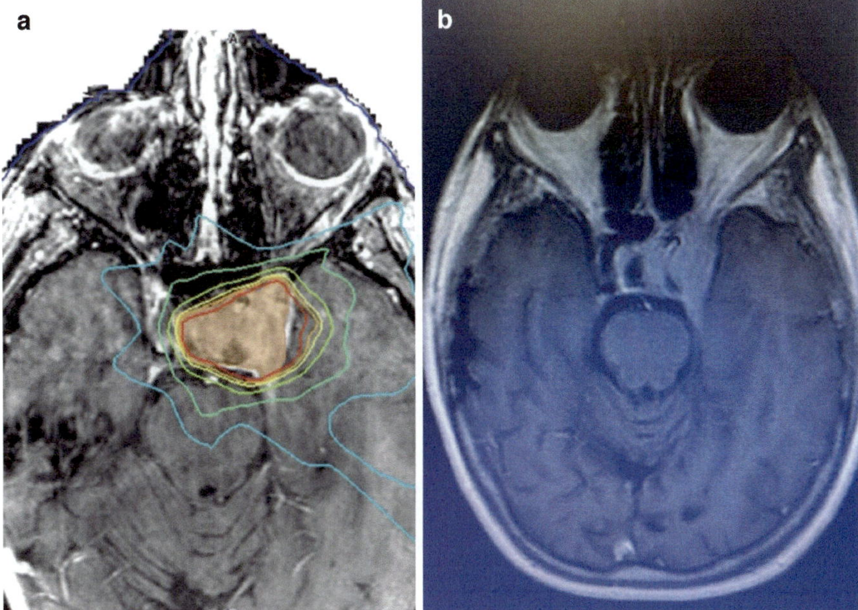

Fig. 14.2 This is a 72-year-old woman found to have an incidental left cavernous sinus meningioma that was enlarging (**a**). She was otherwise healthy. She underwent hypofractionated radiosurgery treatment performed over five sessions. Six years later, the tumor remained stable, and she remained neurologically intact (**b**)

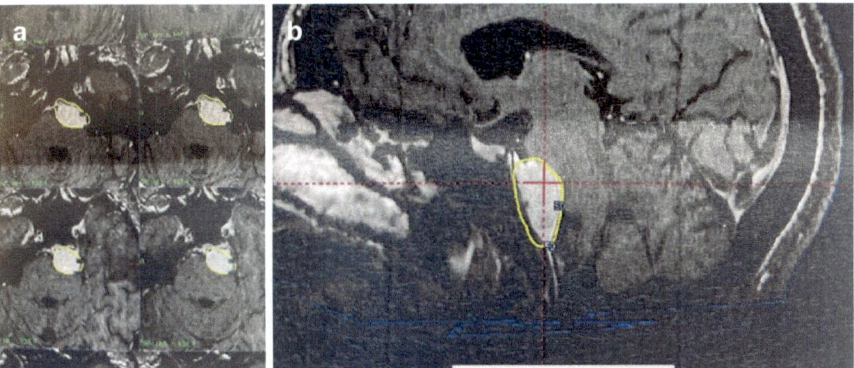

Fig. 14.3 This is a 67-year-old man incidentally discovered to have a moderate sized petroclival meningioma. He was treated uneventfully with Gamma Knife (**a**: axial MRI postcontrast images from the day of Gamma Knife treatment; **b**: sagittal MRI postcontrast image from the day of Gamma Knife treatment)

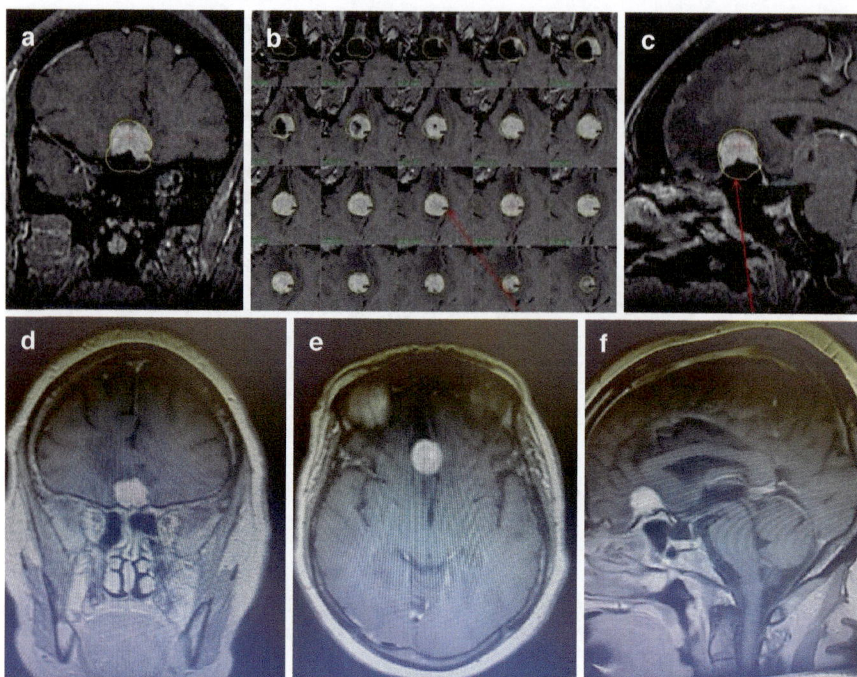

Fig. 14.4 This is a 60-year-old woman found incidentally to have a planum sphenoidale meningioma with a calcified base and some edema. The patient was treated with Gamma Knife (**a**: postcontrast T1 coronal MRI image at the time of Gamma Knife treatment; **b**: postcontrast T1 axial MRI images at the time of Gamma Knife treatment; **c**: postcontrast sagittal MRI images at the time of Gamma Knife treatment). Four years later, the patient had no symptoms, and the tumor remained stable (**d**: postcontrast T1 coronal MRI image; **e**: postcontrast T1 axial MRI image; **f**: postcontrast T1 sagittal MRI image)

Chapter 15
Encephaloceles and Spontaneous CSF Leaks

A separate subcategory of skull base surgery problems in adults that may need to be addressed surgically are frontal and temporal encephaloceles.

The frontal lobe may erode through the floor of the anterior skull base and cause CSF leakage. If this occurs, surgical repair is appropriate. This can usually be best accomplished with a transnasal endoscopic approach [87] with concomitant placement of a lumbar drain (for 2–3 days) rather than the more invasive craniotomy (see Fig. 15.1).

The temporal lobe may also erode through the temporal bone allowing leakage of CSF into the temporal bone air cells. If the tympanic membrane is perforated, this can lead to CSF otorrhea. If the tympanic membrane is intact, this can lead to ipsilateral hearing loss or CSF rhinorrhea. Such temporal lobe encephaloceles and dural defects can be treated with a small temporal craniotomy with an extradural repair of the underside of the temporal dura [88]. Chances of successful repair are increased with intraoperative placement of a lumbar drain, left in for 2–3 days (see Fig. 15.2).

M. H. Brisman, *Put Down the Knife*,
https://doi.org/10.1007/978-3-031-48499-5_15

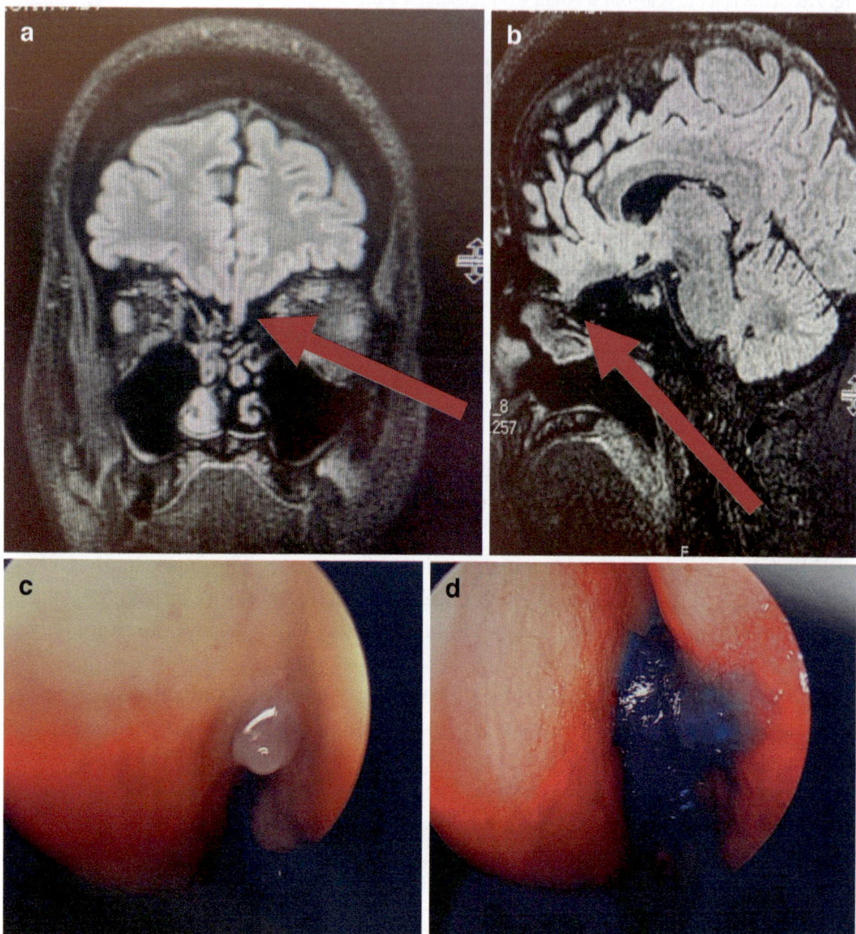

Fig. 15.1 This is a 36-year-old man with recent drainage of clear fluid from his left nostril. Testing demonstrated CSF. MRI imaging demonstrated an encephalocele at the anterior left skull base (**a**: coronal flair MRI; **b**: sagittal flair MRI). He underwent endonasal endoscopic allograft repair through the left nostril with concurrent placement of a lumbar drain for 2 days (**c**: intra-operative view of the defect with CSF leaking; **d**: intra-operative view after the repair). Subsequently, the patient did well, and the leaking stopped

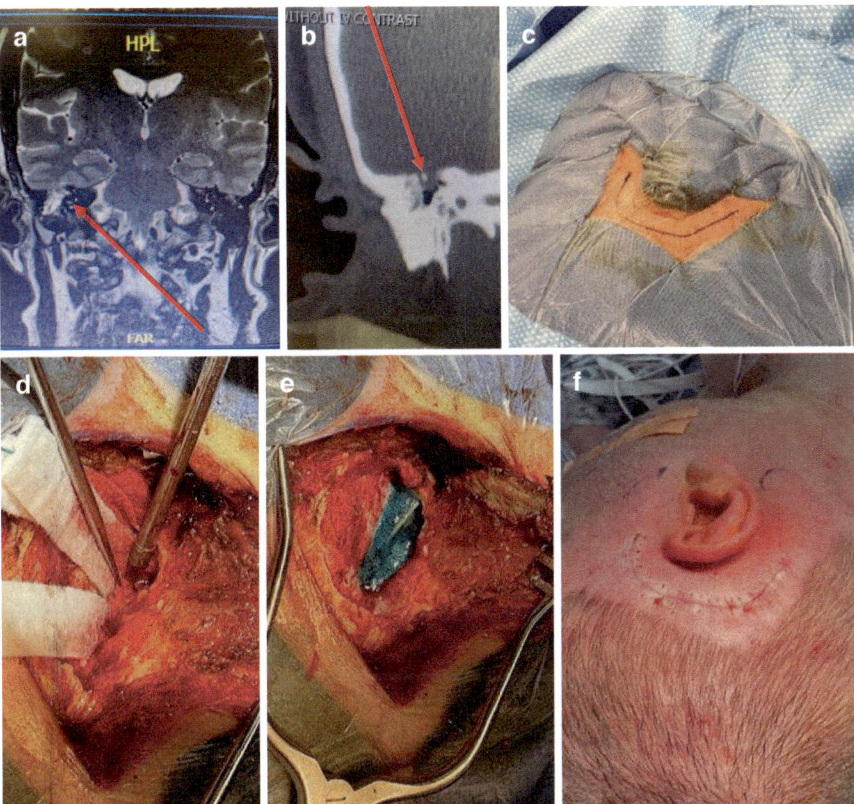

Fig. 15.2 This is a 48-year-old man who had several months of clogged hearing in the right ear. Imaging was consistent with a temporal encephalocele eroding into the mastoid air cells (**a**: T2 weighted coronal MRI image; **b**: CT skull window coronal image). The patient underwent a small right temporal craniotomy and repair of the defect with an extradural approach using allograft material and a lumbar drain for 2 days (**c**: intraoperative incision planned above the right ear; **d**: intraoperative exposure of the subtemporal dura and the bony defect; **e**: intraoperative allograft repair; **f**: closed incision at end of surgery). The patient did well, and after several months his hearing had returned to normal

Chapter 16
Epilepsy

Seizures are sometimes caused by a discrete brain lesion, the removal of which may eliminate the seizures. Also, there are now many seizure medicines that are very effective and well-tolerated. Levetiracetam/Keppra is often used now as the first line medical treatment for seizures. Levetiracetam and lamotrigine are considered to be two of the safest anti-seizure medicines for use during pregnancy. "Epilepsy surgery" usually refers to surgery for seizures in which there is no clear anatomical brain lesion causing the seizures and the seizures are refractory to medicines. The need for such surgery is rare. Various surface and internal electrodes may help localize the seizure focus. The most common type of surgery is for mesial temporal lobe epilepsy (MTLE), in which the mesial temporal lobe is demonstrated to be the cause of the seizures. These patients can be treated with either temporal lobectomy [89] or laser interstitial thermal therapy (LITT) [90]. Other seizure foci beside the temporal lobe can also sometimes be targeted for excision if they are in non-eloquent regions of the brain.

M. H. Brisman, *Put Down the Knife*,
https://doi.org/10.1007/978-3-031-48499-5_16

Chapter 17
Psychosurgery

There was a time not so long ago when psychosurgery (brain surgery for the treatment of psychiatric disorders) was quite common, particularly the frontal lobotomy for the treatment of a wide variety of serious psychiatric disorders. Frontal lobotomy fell out of favor with the advent of better medical treatments for these disorders.

While there may be some surgical procedures still offered for the most severe and medically refractory cases, such as severe depression or severe obsessive-compulsive disorder, these types of procedures are rarely performed today.

M. H. Brisman, *Put Down the Knife*,
https://doi.org/10.1007/978-3-031-48499-5_17

Chapter 18
Non-surgical Management of Neurosurgery Patients

The help that a brain surgeon can provide to a patient goes far beyond brain surgery itself. The significance of the physician–patient encounter cannot be overemphasized. Many patients, given the significance of the interaction, will always remember the time they were seen by a brain surgeon, even if it is just for a single visit that never results in any surgery.

The surgeon should try their very best to be on time for their visit. Just like being on time is a universal sign of respect, being late is a universal sign of disrespect. Obviously in this line of work, emergencies can always develop, and if they do, the surgeon should apologize, and patients will usually understand. But all efforts should be made to see patients at the scheduled time. And, as my mother always said, the secret to always being on time is being early. Furthermore, the surgeon should have enough time set aside to reasonably address each patient's needs.

The surgeon should make sure that both they and the patient are optimally prepared so as to make the most of the visit time. Any relevant images, blood work, testing, paperwork, doctors' records, and other materials should be obtained and reviewed if possible before the visit so the time spent will be most useful for the patient. Basic clinical information written in layman's terms can also be sent to the patient to review beforehand if that would be helpful.

The surgeon should always begin by listening to what the patient has come there to say. Some of this information may be critical in deciding if the person needs brain surgery. Some of this information may not be necessary for the surgical decision itself but may be very important for the patient to express. Patients often feel better just from expressing their health concerns and being fully heard out. Furthermore, listening to all of a patient's concerns is important in establishing a proper physician–patient relationship. The patient must feel comfortable in expressing anything they feel may be important and in knowing that the surgeon will listen seriously to any such concerns, as neither the surgeon nor the patient know in advance all the possible things that may or may not be important to be communicated to the surgeon.

M. H. Brisman, *Put Down the Knife*,
https://doi.org/10.1007/978-3-031-48499-5_18

The surgeon should explain what he or she thinks is the problem and the options for treating it. Risks, benefits, and alternatives of all reasonable options should be presented. In general, brain surgery should be recommended only if absolutely necessary, and even then, offering lower risk procedures should be the rule. It is rarely appropriate to offer something that will make the patient worse off. The surgeon should usually be offering patients what they would want for themselves or their own family members.

The surgeon should be prepared to follow the patient without surgery until such time as it may become clear that surgery would or would not be most appropriate. Further testing may first be appropriate. Medical management or other conservative measures might be an appropriate first option. The patient and family may need time to consider things. Most patients seen in the office will not need emergency surgery. The patient and family should have easy access to the surgeon to discuss any treatment or surgery they are considering. I always give patients my cell phone number.

It is important to give patients hope. Even when circumstances seem most unfortunate, a message of hope is always important for both patients and their families.

If an operation is performed, it is critical to follow the patients closely to make sure an optimal outcome will be obtained. This includes regularly visiting the patient in person while in the hospital and frequently communicating with the patient and their family. Patients must feel comfortable expressing any possible concern to their surgeon after surgery.

Patients who are seen by adult brain surgeons will often also have physical distress (such as cranio-facial pain) or emotional distress (e.g., stress, anxiety, or depressed mood) related to their brain problem/brain surgery problem. There are many non-surgical interventions that can be very helpful to such patients. While there are often other professionals who can assist with these issues, sometimes there are not, and sometimes the neurosurgeon is in the best position to try to help the patient with these problems. These non-surgical remedies are often not focused on.

It is also important to recognize that "pain" and other upsetting feelings are influenced by many different factors including mood, anxiety, stress, and social support. Pain may also have peripheral nerve generators, central brain generators, or muscular generators. As such, a multimodal approach is often best for more difficult to treat cases. Also, it is important to keep in mind that many pain or other problems will improve with time.

Below are options for the management of cranio-facial pain problems (I give patients a printed copy of these possible options).

Non-medical, Non-invasive Treatments

- Addressing depressed mood: Anything that can be done to help with a person's mood and avoid a depressed mood can be helpful. Sometimes just letting patients know that there are many options available and that there is good reason for hope can improve how a patient feels. An internist, psychologist, or psychiatrist might also be helpful here.

- Addressing anxiety: Anything that can be done to alleviate a patient's anxiety can also help. Sometimes just taking the time to rule out other diseases and giving the patient reassurance about their condition may be helpful. Letting the patient understand that the condition may well improve with time may also help. Therapists might also be able to help here.
- Addressing stress: Anything that can be done to lessen a patient's stress levels can help. Often other family members need to be more sensitive to the patient's pain condition or other medical problems and help them at home so their stress levels are less.
- Meditation or yoga: Sometimes these low risk techniques can help a person better manage their physical and emotional problems.
- Addressing support: Anything that can improve a patient's support structure can help. Support structures can include not only just family and other treating physicians but also include support groups. Some of these are available online. These groups let people share their experiences, discuss things that worked for them, and help people know that they are not alone.
- Application of hot or cold to the painful areas. Sometimes patients may experience relief from periodic application of hot things (like a warm washcloth or a heating pad) or cold things (like an icepack wrapped in a towel) to the face or head. In some cases, these treatments may ease the pain the patient is experiencing.
- Massage treatments/physical therapy: Such treatments can be performed by family members, massage therapists, or physical therapists. Some patients may find this helpful.
- Hypnosis: This is a low risk, non-invasive treatment that may provide moderate pain relief for certain individuals who are susceptible to hypnosis. Such benefits will usually require multiple sessions.

Medical Management

- Over the counter (OTC) pain medicines
  - Tylenol (acetaminophen) is an effective pain reliever for mild to moderate pain.
  - Non-steroidals can also be effective for mild to moderate pain. These include common medicines like aspirin (acetylsalicylic acid), Advil/Motrin (ibuprofen), and Aleve (naproxen sodium). Excedrin is another commonly used medicine that contains aspirin (a non-steroidal) as well as acetaminophen and caffeine.
  - Numbing medicines: Sometimes people may benefit from topical, over the counter numbing medicines like benzocaine, which can be used as a topical pain reliever in the mouth (e.g., Oragel), as a throat lozenge (e.g., Cepacol), or as a skin cream (e.g., Lanacane).

- Antiseizure medicines (anticonvulsants)
  - Neurontin (gabapentin) and Lyrica (pregabalin) are usually the first choice for idiopathic and traumatic neuropathic pain, particularly achy, constant pain. People usually start with gabapentin because it is usually less expensive. These drugs are usually the second-choice medicines for trigeminal neuralgia and glossopharyngeal neuralgia.
  - Tegretol (carbamazepine) and Trileptal (oxcarbazepine) are the first-choice medicines for trigeminal neuralgia and glossopharyngeal neuralgia. They can also be effective for occipital neuralgia. Both medicines can cause some hyponatremia, particularly at higher doses. These medicines can also be useful if there is a "sharp" component to any type of neuropathic cranio-facial pain. Dosing is titrated not based on therapeutic blood levels but rather on pain relief and the development of side effects. Lower dosing is usually needed for older patients.
  - Topamax (topiramate) is another antiseizure medicine that may help with various cranio-facial pain syndromes and headache syndromes.
  - Depakote (sodium valproate) is another antiseizure medicine that may be used after other medicines have been tried. It can also help prevent migraine headaches.
  - Lamictal (lamotrigine) is another antiseizure medicine that may be used after other medicines have been tried.
  - Dilantin (phenytoin) is a useful medicine particularly for people who have responded to antiseizure medicines in the past and need an urgent escalation of antiseizure medicine with some other agent. For example, for patients with trigeminal neuralgia who are maxed out on carbamazepine and gabapentin and come into the emergency room with extreme uncontrolled pain, an intravenous loading dose of Dilantin can often provide relief.
- Anti-Depressants
  - Elavil (amitriptyline) is a tricyclic antidepressant that is also one of the first-choice medicines for chronic neuropathic pain. It is usually taken once a day before bedtime. After gabapentin, Elavil is often the second-choice prescription medicine for refractory neuropathic pain. Elavil should be avoided, if possible, in the elderly.
  - Cymbalta (duloxetine) is a serotonin and norepinephrine reuptake inhibitor (SNRI). It can also be effective for alleviating neuropathic pain.
  - Other anti-depressants can also be used, particularly for treating a patient's depression.
- Anti-inflammatories
  - Steroids can help reduce inflammation and are the first choice for certain inflammatory cranio-facial pain conditions, such as temporal arteritis. However, long-term use has significant side effects. A 1-week course of steroids, such as with a Medrol Dosepak (a tapering dose of methylpredniso-

lone), may be worth trying for patients with neuropathic cranio-facial pain to see if there is a response. If there is, the short-term course of steroids can be used for flare-ups, or, in exceptional cases, a long-term use can be considered but only at very low doses. A positive response to steroids might also suggest an alternate diagnosis.
    - Indomethacin is a prescription non-steroidal anti-inflammatory that is the treatment of choice for paroxysmal hemicrania. It may also be helpful for other types of refractory severe facial pain syndromes.

- Prescription topical pain creams: These creams contain multiple ingredients and are therefore often referred to as "compound pain creams." These are a low-risk option to consider for patients who continue to suffer from significant pain.
- Skeletal muscle relaxants: Lioresal (baclofen), Flexiril (cyclobenzaprine), and Robaxin (methocarbamol). Sometimes, chronic pain syndromes have a significant component of muscle spasm or muscle related pain. For this reason, sometimes muscle relaxants can be helpful. These medicines are addictive, so they should only be used if needed, and ideally for short periods. If they are used for a prolonged period, patients would need to taper them off gradually if a time came when they were no longer necessary.
- Benzodiazepines: Valium (diazepam), Klonopin (clonazepam), Xanax (alprazolam). These medicines have sedative, anti-anxiety, and muscle relaxant properties. This category of medicine is also habit forming and should be used only in very refractory cases of chronic pain. These medicines can help through muscle relaxation, as well as reduction of stressful feelings, tension, and anxiety that often contribute to a chronic pain condition. Again, ideally if these medicines are used at all, they would be used for a short period. Also, when coming off these medicines, a gradual tapering is needed.
- Barbiturates: Butalbital. This is most often used as a component of the medicine Fioricet (butalbital/acetaminophen/caffeine). Fioricet is sometimes used for cranio-facial pain syndromes. However, anything containing barbiturates can also be habit forming. Ideally this could be tried for just a short period if other options fail.
- Marijuana/Cannabis: The main active ingredients in marijuana are tetrahydrocannabinol (THC) and cannabidiol (CBD). While there are definitely downsides to the use of marijuana, for some patients with chronic, refractory pain, this may be considered to try to make the pain less bothersome. Marijuana can be consumed in edible form (such as "gummies") and can also potentiate the effects of other medicines, like gabapentin.
- Ketamine: Ketamine is an anesthetic agent which in low doses might help with severe chronic neuropathic pain, particularly if it is associated with severe depression. It can be dispensed in lozenge forms (troches) or as a nasal spray. Ketamine is addictive and should be administered only under the care of pain specialists.
- Opioids: Tramadol, Oxycontin, Dilaudid, Nucynta. Opioids are really the absolute last resort medicine for the management of chronic pain. They are highly

addictive and subject to abuse. The preferred use of opioids for chronic neuropathic pain, if used at all, is for a rare severe "flare up" of the pain. Opioids are also a reasonable choice for severe neuropathic pain in patients with limited life expectancy, for example, with pain related to end-stage cancer. Opioids are often not an effective treatment for most people with chronic neuropathic pain. That having been said, it is possible that there is a small subgroup of people with chronic severe neuropathic pain that is refractory to all other measures who might benefit from opioids. There is also evidence that low dose naltrexone (LDN) may also be helpful in the management of refractory chronic neuropathic pain. Patients who are being managed on long-term opioids for chronic pain are usually under the care of a pain management specialist.

Procedures

- Acupuncture: Some people find that this can be helpful, although multiple treatments are usually required.
- Nerve blocks: Sometimes people may experience some relief from various "nerve blocks." These are usually injections of numbing medicines (like lidocaine), steroids, or both. If these do help, they are often short-lived. They may need to be repeated, and it is possible that sometimes these injections can "break the pain cycle." Sometimes, a nerve block may also convey useful information for treating the pain, that is, does the pain respond to temporarily blocking a particular nerve? This may be useful information in terms of other future treatments.
- Botox injections: Botulinum toxin, when used in very tiny doses in a very superficial manner, can cause temporary weakness of various muscles. Because some neuropathic pain is mediated by subtle muscle spasm or tension, Botox may therefore help with some chronic pain syndromes. It may have to be repeated every few months, as the effects are not permanent. Also, Botox may act to relieve chronic pain in other ways that are not fully understood. Regardless, this is a low-risk intervention that can help with certain cranio-facial pain syndromes. It can take 1–2 weeks to give pain relief.
- Peripheral neuro-stimulators: These are very small soft wire electrodes that can be placed under the skin to stimulate various peripheral nerves, such as the supraorbital nerve (the sensory nerve above the eye), the infraorbital nerve (the sensory nerve below the eye), and the occipital nerves (the sensory nerves in the back of the head). The implant takes only a few minutes to place and is then attached to an external power supply and regulator for a few days that allows the patient to adjust the settings to see if the electrode is helping. If it does help, an electrode can then be placed on a more permanent basis and attached to a battery that is internalized under the collarbone, like a pacemaker battery. This is a minimally invasive procedure that can help some people with chronic severe neuro-

pathic cranio-facial pain. Patients who are candidates for this procedure have pain that has lasted at least 6 months and have failed multiple other treatments.

- Hyperbaric oxygen therapy (HBOT): This treatment involves exposing patients to high levels of oxygen under increased pressure in special chambers. The treatments usually are done over several weeks. The higher oxygen levels are thought to enhance healing of tissues. It is unclear whether certain patients with refractory cranio-facial pain might benefit from this or not. (There is evidence that this treatment may help with radiation related injuries, so it would be reasonable to investigate, for example, whether this treatment might help patients with deafferentation pain that occurred after a radiosurgery treatment for trigeminal neuralgia.)
- Ketamine infusions: Ketamine is an anesthetic. When administered in low infusion doses, it may help to reduce the pain associated with some chronic cranio-facial pain syndromes. Several outpatient treatments are required. There may be a role for this treatment in patients who have chronic cranio-facial pain, particularly if it is associated with severe refractory depression (which ketamine infusions can also help).

There are many options for treating cranio-facial pain and the distressing problems that often accompany brain problems and brain surgery problems. These mostly involve medicines and non-surgical treatments. For refractory cases, there are some procedures that may offer relief. Treating physicians must be very patient and willing to try a host of treatments for these often difficult to manage cases. The best chance of success comes with a willingness to try different treatments, including multiple medicines at different doses and treatments in different combinations. Multimodality efforts (using multiple treatments options) are usually more likely to succeed. The role of the brain surgeon in the diagnosis and management of these disorders is complementary to the role of other specialists, including family practice doctors, internists, neurologists, ophthalmologists, otolaryngologists, pain management doctors, dentists, physiatrists, psychologists, psychiatrists, and social workers.

Conclusion

Only a small percent of the adult population will benefit from brain surgery. Of those who will, most will benefit from a less invasive, smaller, and focused procedure, performed by an experienced brain surgeon. Recent technological advances have made adult brain surgery safer than it has ever been in the modern era. Experienced adult brain surgeons are the ones who should be making the decisions in regards to adult brain surgery. Many brain operations currently being performed should be reconsidered, in favor of less invasive procedures or non-surgical options.

M. H. Brisman, *Put Down the Knife*, https://doi.org/10.1007/978-3-031-48499-5

References

1. Kwok AC, Semel ME, Lipsitz SR, Bader AM, Barnato AE, Gawande AA, Jha AK. The intensity and variation of surgical care at the end of life: a retrospective cohort study. Lancet. 2011;378(9800):1408–13.
2. Nabozny MJ, Kruser JM, Steffens NM, Brasel KJ, Campbell TC, Gaines ME, Schwarze ML. Constructing high-stakes surgical decisions: it's better to die trying. Ann Surg. 2016;263(1):64–70.
3. Knowing when not to operate. BMJ. 1999;318:0.
4. Makoshi Z, Toop N, Smith LGF, Drapeau A, Pindrik J, Sribnick EA, Leonard J, Shaikhouni A. Association between synthetic sealants and increased complication rates in posterior fossa decompression with duraplasty for Chiari malformations regardless of graft type. J Neurosurg Pediatr. 2022:1–10.
5. Meyer HS, Wagner A, Obermueller T, Negwer C, Wostrack M, Krieg S, Gempt J, Meyer B. Assessment of the incidence and nature of adverse events and their association with human error in neurosurgery. A prospective observation. Brain Spine. 2021;2:100853.
6. Bates DW, Levine DM, Salmasian H, Syrowatka A, Shahian DM, Lipsitz S, Zebrowski JP, Myers LC, Logan MS, Roy CG, Iannaccone C, Frits ML, Volk LA, Dulgarian S, Amato MG, Edrees HH, Sato L, Folcarelli P, Einbinder JS, Reynolds ME, Mort E. The safety of inpatient health care. N Engl J Med. 2023;388(2):142–53.
7. Hanley DF, Thompson RE, Rosenblum M, Yenokyan G, Lane K, McBee N, Mayo SW, Bistran-Hall AJ, Gandhi D, Mould WA, Ullman N, Ali H, Carhuapoma JR, Kase CS, Lees KR, Dawson J, Wilson A, Betz JF, Sugar EA, Hao Y, Avadhani R, Caron JL, Harrigan MR, Carlson AP, Bulters D, LeDoux D, Huang J, Cobb C, Gupta G, Kitagawa R, Chicoine MR, Patel H, Dodd R, Camarata PJ, Wolfe S, Stadnik A, Money PL, Mitchell P, Sarabia R, Harnof S, Barzo P, Unterberg A, Teitelbaum JS, Wang W, Anderson CS, Mendelow AD, Gregson B, Janis S, Vespa P, Ziai W, Zuccarello M, Awad IA, MISTIE III Investigators. Efficacy and safety of minimally invasive surgery with thrombolysis in intracerebral haemorrhage evacuation (MISTIE III): a randomised, controlled, open-label, blinded endpoint phase 3 trial. Lancet. 2019;393(10175):1021–32.
8. Mohr JP, Parides MK, Stapf C, Moquete E, Moy CS, Overbey JR, Al-Shahi Salman R, Vicaut E, Young WL, Houdart E, Cordonnier C, Stefani MA, Hartmann A, von Kummer R, Biondi A, Berkefeld J, Klijn CJ, Harkness K, Libman R, Barreau X, Moskowitz AJ, International ARUBA Investigators. Medical management with or without interventional therapy for unruptured brain arteriovenous malformations (ARUBA): a multicentre, non-blinded, randomised trial. Lancet. 2014;383(9917):614–21.

M. H. Brisman, *Put Down the Knife*, https://doi.org/10.1007/978-3-031-48499-5

9. Peres CMA, Caldas JGMP, Puglia P, de Andrade AF, da Silva IAF, Teixeira MJ, Figueiredo EG. Endovascular management of acute epidural hematomas: clinical experience with 80 cases. J Neurosurg. 2018;128(4):1044–50.
10. van Essen TA, van Erp IAM, Lingsma HF, Pisică D, Yue JK, Singh RD, van Dijck JTJM, Volovici V, Younsi A, Kolias A, Peppel LD, Heijenbrok-Kal M, Ribbers GM, Menon DK, Hutchinson PJA, Manley GT, Depreitere B, Steyerberg EW, Maas AIR, de Ruiter GCW, Peul WC, CENTER-TBI Investigators and Participants. Comparative effectiveness of decompressive craniectomy versus craniotomy for traumatic acute subdural hematoma (CENTER-TBI): an observational cohort study. EClinicalMedicine. 2023;63:102161.
11. Kageyama H, Toyooka T, Tsuzuki N, Oka K. Nonsurgical treatment of chronic subdural hematoma with tranexamic acid. J Neurosurg. 2013;119(2):332–7.
12. Kutty RK, Leela SK, Sreemathyamma SB, Sivanandapanicker JL, Asher P, Peethambaran A, Prabhakar RB. The outcome of medical management of chronic subdural hematoma with tranexamic acid—a prospective observational study. J Stroke Cerebrovasc Dis. 2020;29(11):105273.
13. Joyce E, Bounajem MT, Scoville J, Thomas AJ, Ogilvy CS, Riina HA, Tanweer O, Levy EI, Spiotta AM, Gross BA, Jankowitz BT, Cawley CM, Khalessi AA, Pandey AS, Ringer AJ, Hanel R, Ortiz RA, Langer D, Levitt MR, Binning M, Taussky P, Kan P, Grandhi R. Middle meningeal artery embolization treatment of nonacute subdural hematomas in the elderly: a multiinstitutional experience of 151 cases. Neurosurg Focus. 2020;49(4):E5.
14. Kan P, Maragkos GA, Srivatsan A, Srinivasan V, Johnson J, Burkhardt JK, Robinson TM, Salem MM, Chen S, Riina HA, Tanweer O, Levy EI, Spiotta AM, Kasab SA, Lena J, Gross BA, Cherian J, Cawley CM, Howard BM, Khalessi AA, Pandey AS, Ringer AJ, Hanel R, Ortiz RA, Langer D, Kelly CM, Jankowitz BT, Ogilvy CS, Moore JM, Levitt MR, Binning M, Grandhi R, Siddiq F, Thomas AJ. Middle meningeal artery embolization for chronic subdural hematoma: a multi-center experience of 154 consecutive embolizations. Neurosurgery. 2021;88(2):268–77.
15. Mendelow AD, Gregson BA, Fernandes HM, Murray GD, Teasdale GM, Hope DT, Karimi A, Shaw MD, Barer DH, STICH Investigators. Early surgery versus initial conservative treatment in patients with spontaneous supratentorial intracerebral haematomas in the International Surgical Trial in Intracerebral Haemorrhage (STICH): a randomised trial. Lancet. 2005;365(9457):387–97.
16. Mendelow AD, Gregson BA, Rowan EN, Murray GD, Gholkar A, Mitchell PM, STICH II Investigators. Early surgery versus initial conservative treatment in patients with spontaneous supratentorial lobar intracerebral haematomas (STICH II): a randomised trial. Lancet. 2013;382(9890):397–408.
17. Gregson BA, Rowan EN, Francis R, McNamee P, Boyers D, Mitchell P, McColl E, Chambers IR, Unterberg A, Mendelow AD, STITCH(TRAUMA) Investigators. Surgical Trial In Traumatic intraCerebral Haemorrhage (STITCH): a randomised controlled trial of Early Surgery compared with Initial Conservative Treatment. Health Technol Assess. 2015;19(70):1–138.
18. Kuramatsu JB, Biffi A, Gerner ST, Sembill JA, Sprügel MI, Leasure A, Sansing L, Matouk C, Falcone GJ, Endres M, Haeusler KG, Sobesky J, Schurig J, Zweynert S, Bauer M, Vajkoczy P, Ringleb PA, Purrucker J, Rizos T, Volkmann J, Müllges W, Kraft P, Schubert AL, Erbguth F, Nueckel M, Schellinger PD, Glahn J, Knappe UJ, Fink GR, Dohmen C, Stetefeld H, Fisse AL, Minnerup J, Hagemann G, Rakers F, Reichmann H, Schneider H, Rahmig J, Ludolph AC, Stösser S, Neugebauer H, Röther J, Michels P, Schwarz M, Reimann G, Bäzner H, Schwert H, Claßen J, Michalski D, Grau A, Palm F, Urbanek C, Wöhrle JC, Alshammari F, Horn M, Bahner D, Witte OW, Günther A, Hamann GF, Hagen M, Roeder SS, Lücking H, Dörfler A, Testai FD, Woo D, Schwab S, Sheth KN, Huttner HB. Association of surgical hematoma evacuation vs conservative treatment with functional outcome in patients with cerebellar intracerebral hemorrhage. JAMA. 2019;322(14):1392–403.

19. Singh SD, Brouwers HB, Senff JR, Pasi M, Goldstein J, Viswanathan A, Klijn CJM, Rinkel GJE. Haematoma evacuation in cerebellar intracerebral haemorrhage: systematic review. J Neurol Neurosurg Psychiatry. 2020;91(1):82–7.
20. Hanley DF, Lane K, McBee N, Ziai W, Tuhrim S, Lees KR, Dawson J, Gandhi D, Ullman N, Mould WA, Mayo SW, Mendelow AD, Gregson B, Butcher K, Vespa P, Wright DW, Kase CS, Carhuapoma JR, Keyl PM, Diener-West M, Muschelli J, Betz JF, Thompson CB, Sugar EA, Yenokyan G, Janis S, John S, Harnof S, Lopez GA, Aldrich EF, Harrigan MR, Ansari S, Jallo J, Caron JL, LeDoux D, Adeoye O, Zuccarello M, Adams HP Jr, Rosenblum M, Thompson RE, Awad IA, CLEAR III Investigators. Thrombolytic removal of intraventricular haemorrhage in treatment of severe stroke: results of the randomised, multicentre, multiregion, placebo-controlled CLEAR III trial. Lancet. 2017;389(10069):603–11.
21. Molyneux AJ, Kerr RS, Yu LM, Clarke M, Sneade M, Yarnold JA, Sandercock P, International Subarachnoid Aneurysm Trial (ISAT) Collaborative Group. International subarachnoid aneurysm trial (ISAT) of neurosurgical clipping versus endovascular coiling in 2143 patients with ruptured intracranial aneurysms: a randomised comparison of effects on survival, dependency, seizures, rebleeding, subgroups, and aneurysm occlusion. Lancet. 2005;366(9488):809–17.
22. International Study of Unruptured Intracranial Aneurysms Investigators. Unruptured intracranial aneurysms—risk of rupture and risks of surgical intervention. N Engl J Med. 1998;339(24):1725–33. https://doi.org/10.1056/NEJM199812103392401. Erratum in: N Engl J Med 1999 Mar 4;340(9):744.
23. Wiebers DO, Whisnant JP, Huston J 3rd, Meissner I, Brown RD Jr, Piepgras DG, Forbes GS, Thielen K, Nichols D, O'Fallon WM, Peacock J, Jaeger L, Kassell NF, Kongable-Beckman GL, Torner JC, International Study of Unruptured Intracranial Aneurysms Investigators. Unruptured intracranial aneurysms: natural history, clinical outcome, and risks of surgical and endovascular treatment. Lancet. 2003;362(9378):103–10.
24. Koyanagi M, Ishii A, Imamura H, Satow T, Yoshida K, Hasegawa H, Kikuchi T, Takenobu Y, Ando M, Takahashi JC, Nakahara I, Sakai N, Miyamoto S. Long-term outcomes of coil embolization of unruptured intracranial aneurysms. J Neurosurg. 2018;129(6):1492–8.
25. Starke RM, Kano H, Ding D, Lee JY, Mathieu D, Whitesell J, Pierce JT, Huang PP, Kondziolka D, Yen CP, Feliciano C, Rodgriguez-Mercado R, Almodovar L, Pieper DR, Grills IS, Silva D, Abbassy M, Missios S, Barnett GH, Lunsford LD, Sheehan JP. Stereotactic radiosurgery for cerebral arteriovenous malformations: evaluation of long-term outcomes in a multicenter cohort. J Neurosurg. 2017;126(1):36–44.
26. Mohr JP, Overbey JR, Hartmann A, Kummer RV, Al-Shahi Salman R, Kim H, van der Worp HB, Parides MK, Stefani MA, Houdart E, Libman R, Pile-Spellman J, Harkness K, Cordonnier C, Moquete E, Biondi A, Klijn CJM, Stapf C, Moskowitz AJ, ARUBA Co-investigators. Medical management with interventional therapy versus medical management alone for unruptured brain arteriovenous malformations (ARUBA): final follow-up of a multicentre, non-blinded, randomised controlled trial. Lancet Neurol. 2020;19(7):573–81.
27. Al-Shahi Salman R, White PM, Counsell CE, du Plessis J, van Beijnum J, Josephson CB, Wilkinson T, Wedderburn CJ, Chandy Z, St George EJ, Sellar RJ, Warlow CP, Scottish Audit of Intracranial Vascular Malformations Collaborators. Outcome after conservative management or intervention for unruptured brain arteriovenous malformations. JAMA. 2014;311(16):1661–9.
28. Wen R, Shi Y, Gao Y, Xu Y, Xiong B, Li D, Gong F, Wang W. The efficacy of gamma knife radiosurgery for cavernous malformations: a meta-analysis and review. World Neurosurg. 2019;123:371–7.
29. Jovin TG, Chamorro A, Cobo E, de Miquel MA, Molina CA, Rovira A, San Román L, Serena J, Abilleira S, Ribó M, Millán M, Urra X, Cardona P, López-Cancio E, Tomasello A, Castaño C, Blasco J, Aja L, Dorado L, Quesada H, Rubiera M, Hernandez-Pérez M, Goyal M, Demchuk AM, von Kummer R, Gallofré M, Dávalos A, REVASCAT Trial Investigators. Thrombectomy within 8 hours after symptom onset in ischemic stroke. N Engl J Med. 2015;372(24):2296–306.

30. Nogueira RG, Jadhav AP, Haussen DC, Bonafe A, Budzik RF, Bhuva P, Yavagal DR, Ribo M, Cognard C, Hanel RA, Sila CA, Hassan AE, Millan M, Levy EI, Mitchell P, Chen M, English JD, Shah QA, Silver FL, Pereira VM, Mehta BP, Baxter BW, Abraham MG, Cardona P, Veznedaroglu E, Hellinger FR, Feng L, Kirmani JF, Lopes DK, Jankowitz BT, Frankel MR, Costalat V, Vora NA, Yoo AJ, Malik AM, Furlan AJ, Rubiera M, Aghaebrahim A, Olivot JM, Tekle WG, Shields R, Graves T, Lewis RJ, Smith WS, Liebeskind DS, Saver JL, Jovin TG, DAWN Trial Investigators. Thrombectomy 6 to 24 hours after stroke with a mismatch between deficit and infarct. N Engl J Med. 2018;378(1):11–21.
31. Jüttler E, Schwab S, Schmiedek P, Unterberg A, Hennerici M, Woitzik J, Witte S, Jenetzky E, Hacke W, DESTINY Study Group. Decompressive Surgery for the Treatment of Malignant Infarction of the Middle Cerebral Artery (DESTINY): a randomized, controlled trial. Stroke. 2007;38(9):2518–25.
32. Vahedi K, Vicaut E, Mateo J, Kurtz A, Orabi M, Guichard JP, Boutron C, Couvreur G, Rouanet F, Touzé E, Guillon B, Carpentier A, Yelnik A, George B, Payen D, Bousser MG, DECIMAL Investigators. Sequential-design, multicenter, randomized, controlled trial of early decompressive craniectomy in malignant middle cerebral artery infarction (DECIMAL Trial). Stroke. 2007;38(9):2506–17.
33. Hofmeijer J, Kappelle LJ, Algra A, Amelink GJ, van Gijn J, van der Worp HB, HAMLET Investigators. Surgical decompression for space-occupying cerebral infarction (the Hemicraniectomy After Middle Cerebral Artery infarction with Life-threatening Edema Trial [HAMLET]): a multicentre, open, randomised trial. Lancet Neurol. 2009;8(4):326–33.
34. Zhao J, Su YY, Zhang Y, Zhang YZ, Zhao R, Wang L, Gao R, Chen W, Gao D. Decompressive hemicraniectomy in malignant middle cerebral artery infarct: a randomized controlled trial enrolling patients up to 80 years old. Neurocrit Care. 2012;17(2):161–71.
35. Slezins J, Keris V, Bricis R, Millers A, Valeinis E, Stukens J, Minibajeva O. Preliminary results of randomized controlled study on decompressive craniectomy in treatment of malignant middle cerebral artery stroke. Medicina (Kaunas). 2012;48(10):521–4.
36. Frank JI, Schumm LP, Wroblewski K, Chyatte D, Rosengart AJ, Kordeck C, Thisted RA, HeADDFIRST Trialists. Hemicraniectomy and durotomy upon deterioration from infarction-related swelling trial: randomized pilot clinical trial. Stroke. 2014;45(3):781–7.
37. Jüttler E, Unterberg A, Woitzik J, Bösel J, Amiri H, Sakowitz OW, Gondan M, Schiller P, Limprecht R, Luntz S, Schneider H, Pinzer T, Hobohm C, Meixensberger J, Hacke W, DESTINY II Investigators. Hemicraniectomy in older patients with extensive middle-cerebral-artery stroke. N Engl J Med. 2014;370(12):1091–100.
38. Chua AE, Buckley BS, Lapitan MCM, Jamora RDG. Hemicraniectomy for malignant middle cerebral artery infarction (HeMMI): a randomized controlled clinical trial of decompressive hemicraniectomy with standardized medical care versus standardized medical care alone. Acta Med Philip. 2015;49(1):28–33.
39. Alexander P, Heels-Ansdell D, Siemieniuk R, Bhatnagar N, Chang Y, Fei Y, Zhang Y, McLeod S, Prasad K, Guyatt G. Hemicraniectomy versus medical treatment with large MCA infarct: a review and meta-analysis. BMJ Open. 2016;6(11):e014390.
40. Jauss M, Krieger D, Hornig C, Schramm J, Busse O. Surgical and medical management of patients with massive cerebellar infarctions: results of the German-Austrian Cerebellar Infarction Study. J Neurol. 1999;246(4):257–64.
41. Jüttler E, Schweickert S, Ringleb PA, Huttner HB, Köhrmann M, Aschoff A. Long-term outcome after surgical treatment for space-occupying cerebellar infarction: experience in 56 patients. Stroke. 2009;40(9):3060–6.
42. Mostofi K. Neurosurgical management of massive cerebellar infarct outcome in 53 patients. Surg Neurol Int. 2013;4:28.
43. Bullock MR, Chesnut R, Ghajar J, Gordon D, Hartl R, Newell DW, Servadei F, Walters BC, Wilberger J, Surgical Management of Traumatic Brain Injury Author Group. Surgical management of traumatic parenchymal lesions. Neurosurgery. 2006;58(3 Suppl):S25–46.

44. Cremer OL, van Dijk GW, van Wensen E, Brekelmans GJ, Moons KG, Leenen LP, Kalkman CJ. Effect of intracranial pressure monitoring and targeted intensive care on functional outcome after severe head injury. Crit Care Med. 2005;33(10):2207–13.
45. Shafi S, Diaz-Arrastia R, Madden C, Gentilello L. Intracranial pressure monitoring in brain-injured patients is associated with worsening of survival. J Trauma. 2008;64(2):335–40.
46. Chesnut RM, Temkin N, Carney N, Dikmen S, Rondina C, Videtta W, Petroni G, Lujan S, Pridgeon J, Barber J, Machamer J, Chaddock K, Celix JM, Cherner M, Hendrix T, Global Neurotrauma Research Group. A trial of intracranial-pressure monitoring in traumatic brain injury. N Engl J Med. 2012;367(26):2471–81.
47. Volovici V, Pisică D, Gravesteijn BY, et al. Comparative effectiveness of intracranial hypertension management guided by ventricular versus intraparenchymal pressure monitoring: a CENTER-TBI study. Acta Neurochir. 2022;164:1693–705.
48. Banik S, Rath GP, Lamsal R, Sinha S, Bithal PK. Intracranial pressure monitoring in children with severe traumatic brain injury: a retrospective study. J Pediatr Neurosci. 2019;14(1):7–15.
49. Cooper DJ, Rosenfeld JV, Murray L, Arabi YM, Davies AR, D'Urso P, Kossmann T, Ponsford J, Seppelt I, Reilly P, Wolfe R, DECRA Trial Investigators, Australian and New Zealand Intensive Care Society Clinical Trials Group. Decompressive craniectomy in diffuse traumatic brain injury. N Engl J Med. 2011;364(16):1493–502.
50. Hutchinson PJ, Kolias AG, Timofeev IS, Corteen EA, Czosnyka M, Timothy J, Anderson I, Bulters DO, Belli A, Eynon CA, Wadley J, Mendelow AD, Mitchell PM, Wilson MH, Critchley G, Sahuquillo J, Unterberg A, Servadei F, Teasdale GM, Pickard JD, Menon DK, Murray GD, Kirkpatrick PJ, RESCUEicp Trial Collaborators. Trial of decompressive craniectomy for traumatic intracranial hypertension. N Engl J Med. 2016;375(12):1119–30.
51. Deng Y, Li Y, Li X, Wu L, Quan T, Peng C, Fu J, Yang X, Yu J. Long-term results of Gamma Knife Radiosurgery for Postsurgical residual or recurrent nonfunctioning Pituitary Adenomas. Int J Med Sci. 2020;17(11):1532–40.
52. Lee WJ, Cho KR, Choi JW, Kong DS, Seol HJ, Nam DH, Lee JI. Gamma knife radiosurgery as a primary treatment for nonfunctioning pituitary adenoma invading the cavernous sinus. Stereotact Funct Neurosurg. 2020;98(6):371–7.
53. Singh TD, Valizadeh N, Meyer FB, Atkinson JL, Erickson D, Rabinstein AA. Management and outcomes of pituitary apoplexy. J Neurosurg. 2015;122(6):1450–7.
54. Donegan D, Saeed Z, Delivanis DA, Murad MH, Honegger J, Amereller F, Oguz SH, Erickson D, Bancos I. Outcomes of initial management strategies in patients with autoimmune lymphocytic hypophysitis: a systematic review and meta-analysis. J Clin Endocrinol Metab. 2022;107(4):1170–90.
55. Myrseth E, Møller P, Pedersen PH, Lund-Johansen M. Vestibular schwannoma: surgery or gamma knife radiosurgery? A prospective, nonrandomized study. Neurosurgery. 2009;64(4):654–61; discussion 661–3.
56. Jang CK, Jung HH, Chang JH, Chang JW, Park YG, Chang WS. Long-term results of gamma knife radiosurgery for intracranial meningioma. Brain Tumor Res Treat. 2015;3(2):103–7. https://doi.org/10.14791/btrt.2015.3.2.103.
57. Muacevic A, Wowra B, Siefert A, Tonn JC, Steiger HJ, Kreth FW. Microsurgery plus whole brain irradiation versus Gamma Knife surgery alone for treatment of single metastases to the brain: a randomized controlled multicentre phase III trial. J Neurooncol. 2008;87(3):299–307.
58. Wijnenga MMJ, French PJ, Dubbink HJ, Dinjens WNM, Atmodimedjo PN, Kros JM, Smits M, Gahrmann R, Rutten GJ, Verheul JB, Fleischeuer R, Dirven CMF, Vincent AJPE, van den Bent MJ. The impact of surgery in molecularly defined low-grade glioma: an integrated clinical, radiological, and molecular analysis. Neuro Oncol. 2018;20(1):103–12.
59. Tan AC, Ashley DM, López GY, Malinzak M, Friedman HS, Khasraw M. Management of glioblastoma: state of the art and future directions. CA Cancer J Clin. 2020;70(4):299–312.
60. González V, Brell M, Fuster J, Moratinos L, Alegre D, López S, Ibáñez J. Analyzing the role of reoperation in recurrent glioblastoma: a 15-year retrospective study in a single institution. World J Surg Oncol. 2022;20(1):384.

61. Tago M, Terahara A, Shin M, Maruyama K, Kurita H, Nakagawa K, Ohtomo K. Gamma knife surgery for hemangioblastomas. J Neurosurg. 2005;102(Suppl):171–4.
62. Wang C, Liu C, Xiong Y, Han G, Yang H, Wan J, You C. Surgical treatment of intracranial arachnoid cyst in adult patients. Neurol India. 2013;61(1):60–4.
63. Isaacs AM, Ball CG, Hamilton MG. Neuronavigation and laparoscopy guided ventriculo-peritoneal shunt insertion for the treatment of hydrocephalus. J Vis Exp. 2022. https://doi.org/10.3791/62678-v.
64. Hebb AO, Cusimano MD. Idiopathic normal pressure hydrocephalus: a systematic review of diagnosis and outcome. Neurosurgery. 2001;49(5):1166–84; discussion 1184–6.
65. Junkkari A, Häyrinen A, Rauramaa T, Sintonen H, Nerg O, Koivisto AM, Roine RP, Viinamäki H, Soininen H, Luikku A, Jääskeläinen JE, Leinonen V. Health-related quality-of-life outcome in patients with idiopathic normal-pressure hydrocephalus—a 1-year follow-up study. Eur J Neurol. 2017;24(1):58–66.
66. Wu EM, El Ahmadieh TY, Kafka B, Caruso J, Aoun SG, Plitt AR, Neeley O, Olson DM, Ruchinskas RA, Cullum M, Batjer H, White JA. Ventriculoperitoneal shunt outcomes of normal pressure hydrocephalus: a case series of 116 patients. Cureus. 2019;11(3):e4170.
67. Aimard G, Vighetto A, Gabet JY, Bret P, Henry E. Acétazolamide: une alternative à la dérivation dans l'hydrocéphalie à pression normale? Résultats préliminaires [Acetazolamide: an alternative to shunting in normal pressure hydrocephalus? Preliminary results]. Rev Neurol (Paris). 1990;146(6–7):437–9.
68. Alperin N, Oliu CJ, Bagci AM, Lee SH, Kovanlikaya I, Adams D, Katzen H, Ivkovic M, Heier L, Relkin N. Low-dose acetazolamide reverses periventricular white matter hyperintensities in iNPH. Neurology. 2014;82(15):1347–51.
69. Barker FG 2nd, Jannetta PJ, Bissonette DJ, Larkins MV, Jho HD. The long-term outcome of microvascular decompression for trigeminal neuralgia. N Engl J Med. 1996;334(17):1077–83.
70. Kanpolat Y, Savas A, Bekar A, Berk C. Percutaneous controlled radiofrequency trigeminal rhizotomy for the treatment of idiopathic trigeminal neuralgia: 25-year experience with 1,600 patients. Neurosurgery. 2001;48(3):524–32; discussion 532–4.
71. Cheng JS, Lim DA, Chang EF, Barbaro NM. A review of percutaneous treatments for trigeminal neuralgia. Neurosurgery. 2014;10(Suppl 1):25–33; discussion 33.
72. Favoni V, Grimaldi D, Pierangeli G, Cortelli P, Cevoli S. SUNCT/SUNA and neurovascular compression: new cases and critical literature review. Cephalalgia. 2013;33(16):1337–48.
73. Lambru G, Matharu MS. SUNCT, SUNA and trigeminal neuralgia: different disorders or variants of the same disorder? Curr Opin Neurol. 2014;27(3):325–31.
74. Brisman R. Gamma knife radiosurgery for primary management for trigeminal neuralgia. J Neurosurg. 2000;93(Suppl 3):159–61.
75. Kim MK, Park JS, Ahn YH. Microvascular decompression for glossopharyngeal neuralgia: clinical analyses of 30 cases. J Korean Neurosurg Soc. 2017;60(6):738–48.
76. Ellis JA, Mejia Munne JC, Winfree CJ. Trigeminal branch stimulation for the treatment of intractable craniofacial pain. J Neurosurg. 2015;123(1):283–8.
77. Keifer OP Jr, Diaz A, Campbell M, Bezchlibnyk YB, Boulis NM. Occipital nerve stimulation for the treatment of refractory occipital neuralgia: a case series. World Neurosurg. 2017;105:599–604.
78. Hyun SJ, Kong DS, Park K. Microvascular decompression for treating hemifacial spasm: lessons learned from a prospective study of 1,174 operations. Neurosurg Rev. 2010;33(3):325–34; discussion 334.
79. Jo KW, Kong DS, Park K. Microvascular decompression for hemifacial spasm: long-term outcome and prognostic factors, with emphasis on delayed cure. Neurosurg Rev. 2013;36(2):297–301; discussion 301–2.
80. Ohye C, Higuchi Y, Shibazaki T, Hashimoto T, Koyama T, Hirai T, Matsuda S, Serizawa T, Hori T, Hayashi M, Ochiai T, Samura H, Yamashiro K. Gamma knife thalamotomy for Parkinson disease and essential tremor: a prospective multicenter study. Neurosurgery. 2012;70(3):526–35; discussion 535–6.

81. Elias WJ, Lipsman N, Ondo WG, Ghanouni P, Kim YG, Lee W, Schwartz M, Hynynen K, Lozano AM, Shah BB, Huss D, Dallapiazza RF, Gwinn R, Witt J, Ro S, Eisenberg HM, Fishman PS, Gandhi D, Halpern CH, Chuang R, Butts Pauly K, Tierney TS, Hayes MT, Cosgrove GR, Yamaguchi T, Abe K, Taira T, Chang JW. A randomized trial of focused ultrasound thalamotomy for essential tremor. N Engl J Med. 2016;375(8):730–9.
82. Sinai A, Nassar M, Eran A, Constantinescu M, Zaaroor M, Sprecher E, Schlesinger I. Magnetic resonance-guided focused ultrasound thalamotomy for essential tremor: a 5-year single-center experience. J Neurosurg. 2019:1–8.
83. Flora ED, Perera CL, Cameron AL, Maddern GJ. Deep brain stimulation for essential tremor: a systematic review. Mov Disord. 2010;25(11):1550–9.
84. Deuschl G, Schade-Brittinger C, Krack P, Volkmann J, Schäfer H, Bötzel K, Daniels C, Deutschländer A, Dillmann U, Eisner W, Gruber D, Hamel W, Herzog J, Hilker R, Klebe S, Kloss M, Koy J, Krause M, Kupsch A, Lorenz D, Lorenzl S, Mehdorn HM, Moringlane JR, Oertel W, Pinsker MO, Reichmann H, Reuss A, Schneider GH, Schnitzler A, Steude U, Sturm V, Timmermann L, Tronnier V, Trottenberg T, Wojtecki L, Wolf E, Poewe W, Voges J, German Parkinson Study Group, Neurostimulation Section. A randomized trial of deep-brain stimulation for Parkinson's disease. N Engl J Med. 2006;355(9):896–908.
85. Vidailhet M, Vercueil L, Houeto JL, Krystkowiak P, Benabid AL, Cornu P, Lagrange C, Tézenas du Montcel S, Dormont D, Grand S, Blond S, Detante O, Pillon B, Ardouin C, Agid Y, Destée A, Pollak P, French Stimulation du Pallidum Interne dans la Dystonie (SPIDY) Study Group. Bilateral deep-brain stimulation of the globus pallidus in primary generalized dystonia. N Engl J Med. 2005;352(5):459–67.
86. Beecher JS, Liu Y, Qi X, Bolognese PA. Minimally invasive subpial tonsillectomy for Chiari I decompression. Acta Neurochir (Wien). 2016;158(9):1807–11.
87. Nyquist GG, Anand VK, Mehra S, Kacker A, Schwartz TH. Endoscopic endonasal repair of anterior skull base non-traumatic cerebrospinal fluid leaks, meningoceles, and encephaloceles. J Neurosurg. 2010;113(5):961–6.
88. Carlson ML, Copeland WR 3rd, Driscoll CL, Link MJ, Haynes DS, Thompson RC, Weaver KD, Wanna GB. Temporal bone encephalocele and cerebrospinal fluid fistula repair utilizing the middle cranial fossa or combined mastoid-middle cranial fossa approach. J Neurosurg. 2013;119(5):1314–22.
89. Wiebe S, Blume WT, Girvin JP, Eliasziw M, Effectiveness and Efficiency of Surgery for Temporal Lobe Epilepsy Study Group. A randomized, controlled trial of surgery for temporal-lobe epilepsy. N Engl J Med. 2001;345(5):311–8.
90. Le S, Ho AL, Fisher RS, Miller KJ, Henderson JM, Grant GA, Meador KJ, Halpern CH. Laser interstitial thermal therapy (LITT): seizure outcomes for refractory mesial temporal lobe epilepsy. Epilepsy Behav. 2018;89:37–41.

Index

M. H. Brisman, *Put Down the Knife*, https://doi.org/10.1007/978-3-031-48499-5

GPSR Compliance

The European Union's (EU) General Product Safety Regulation (GPSR) is a set of rules that requires consumer products to be safe and our obligations to ensure this.

If you have any concerns about our products, you can contact us on ProductSafety@springernature.com

In case Publisher is established outside the EU, the EU authorized representative is:

Springer Nature Customer Service Center GmbH
Europaplatz 3
69115 Heidelberg, Germany

Batch number: 10370708

Printed by Printforce, the Netherlands